A

M

"Dr. Suzanne Goh is an extraordinary scientist, researcher, and clinician whose pioneering work in autism is changing our thinking about how to best support a child, not only focusing on behavior but also on neurobiology, biochemistry, and physiology. Whether your child is newly diagnosed with autism or you're simply looking for fresh insights and a new way forward, this book is a treasure."

—Dr. Mark Hyman, MD, author of the #1 *New York Times* bestseller *Young Forever*

"Dr. Goh's approach to the care of a child with autism is extraordinarily wise. It considers the whole child—the genetics, biology, family context, interpersonal relationships, cognitive abilities, and emotional life that interact with one another throughout development. This is a much-needed guide for parents and professionals on how best to intervene in ways that will help the child reach his or her greatest potential and experience inner fulfillment."

—Dr. Bradley S. Peterson, MD, director of the Institute for the Developing Mind and chief of Child and Adolescent Psychiatry at Children's Hospital Los Angeles and the Keck School of Medicine, University of Southern California

"In *Magnificent Minds*, Dr. Suzanne Goh presents a refreshing brain-body wholesome biological perspective of autism with timely, practical information for parents and caregivers seeking the best care for autism. It's an essential resource. And I personally love the drawings throughout the book!"

—Dr. Elizabeth Torres, PhD, professor, Rutgers University Department of Psychology, and director of the Sensory Motor Integration Lab

"Wow! This is just the approach the world needs to better understand and support every child with autism."

—Scott Barry Kaufman, PhD, host of *The Psychology Podcast* and author of *Transcend*

"As an autistic adult with multiple co-occurring features, including cerebral palsy, GI issues, and mitochondrial dysfunction, I often struggle with understanding doctors and interacting with the medical system. *Magnificent Minds* presents information clearly and concisely across its well-organized chapters. I found it approachable and learned new things from it as a result, and I expect many others will as well, in a shared journey to better understand and care for the unique autistic people in their lives."

—Jory Fleming, author of *How to Be Human:*
An Autistic Man's Guide to Life

"I wish I had this when Jory was a child."

—Kelly Fleming, mom of Jory Fleming

"Dr. Goh wisely describes a holistic approach to autism that respects that some of the defining characteristics are variations of the human traits that make us uniquely talented. She wants readers to see the whole child for the best results."

—Dr. Mehmet Oz, MD, professor emeritus, Columbia University

"Finally! A well-resourced book that puts it all together for parents and professionals. When a child is diagnosed with autism, parents are bombarded with much information on many levels. The connection between neurobiology, biochemistry, physiology, and the behavioral component is not always clear. Connecting all this to education, community, the importance of family relationships, and possible therapies and what is best for our unique child is difficult for a parent to do. Dr. Goh has explained these complex connections simply, providing hope and fostering the understanding and acceptance of neurodivergence. Certainly, I wish this book had been available when my child was still an infant!"

—Chantal Sicile-Kira, parent, advocate, and author of
What Is Autism?: Understanding Life with Autism or
Asperger's and coauthor of *A Full Life with Autism*

Magnificent Minds

Magnificent Minds

THE NEW WHOLE-CHILD APPROACH TO AUTISM

Dr Suzanne Goh

Vermilion
LONDON

1

Vermilion, an imprint of Ebury Publishing
20 Vauxhall Bridge Road
London SW1V 2SA

Vermilion is part of the Penguin Random House group of companies
whose addresses can be found at global.penguinrandomhouse.com

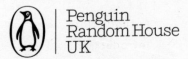

Copyright © 2024 Dr Suzanne Goh

Dr Suzanne Goh has asserted her right to be identified as the author of this
Work in accordance with the Copyright, Designs and Patents Act 1988

First published in Great Britain by Vermilion in 2024
First published in the United States by TarcherPerigee in 2024,
an imprint of Penguin Random House LLC
www.penguin.co.uk

A CIP catalogue record for this book is available from the British Library
Book Design by Laura K.Corless

ISBN: 9781785045103

Printed and bound in Great Britain by Clays Ltd, Elcograf S.p.A.

The authorised representative in the EEA is Penguin Random House Ireland,
Morrison Chambers, 32 Nassau Street, Dublin D02 YH68

Penguin Random House is committed to a sustainable future
for our business, our readers and our planet. This book is made
from Forest Stewardship Council® certified paper.

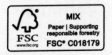

Contents

Author's Note • xi

Introduction • xiii

Part 1 • 1
WHAT AUTISM MEANS

Chapter 1 3
SEEING THE WHOLE CHILD
Understanding *All* of Autism

Chapter 2 23
DIFFERENT, NOT LESS
Embracing Neurodiversity

Chapter 3 35
WHAT'S STRONG WITH ME?
Strengths Outweigh Weaknesses

Chapter 4 47
BEYOND IQ
Recognizing Your Child's Intelligence

Part 2 • 63
THE WHOLE-CHILD PATH

Chapter 5 67
AUTISM PLUS (+)
Improving Brain and Body Health

Chapter 6 121
A DEVELOPMENTAL SYMPHONY
Composing Brain Networks

Chapter 7 183
THE HEART OF BEHAVIOR
ABCs and More

Chapter 8 207
A HAPPY, HEALTHY NEST
Nurturing Your Family

Chapter 9 229
COMMUNITY ADVENTURES
Expanding Your Child's World

Part 3 · 249
LASTING CHANGE

Chapter 10 251
FINDING WISDOM
Lead with the Spirit, the Mind Will Follow

About Cortica · 275

Acknowledgments · 277

Guide to Resources · 281

Glossary of Medical Terms · 287

Notes · 297

Index · 323

About the Author · 333

To all the neurodivergent children and adults I've had the great privilege to know and to their families, thank you for enriching my life and the world we live in. You have been and will always be my greatest teachers.

Author's Note

In this book I use what's called identity-first language (e.g., *autistic child* or *autistic person*), which reflects the preference voiced by autistic self-advocates to view autism as a valued part of one's identity rather than a disorder. Identity-first language represents a shift away from person-first language (e.g., *child with autism* or *person with autism*), which can imply that autism is a disorder that someone "has." Both identity-first and person-first language originated from a desire to emphasize the value and worth of the individual, and both continue to be used widely today. I reserve person-first language for instances when there are multiple diagnoses (e.g., "child with autism, ADHD, and epilepsy" or "person with autism and anxiety").

In this book I use the words *neurodiverse* and *neurodivergent*, which come from the neurodiversity movement. Chapter 2 focuses on neurodiversity and provides more information on how these words are used. Briefly, the word *neurodivergent* refers to individuals who are autistic or who have other neurological differences. The word *neurotypical* refers to non-neurodivergent people. The word *neurodiverse* refers to groups that include people with different neurological characteristics, so a group that includes neurodivergent people, or neurodivergent and neurotypical people, could be called a neurodiverse group.

I use the pronouns *they* and *them* to refer to an individual when the gender identity is unknown.

For people who do not (or do not yet) communicate by speaking, I use the word *nonspeaking* rather than *nonverbal*. The word *nonverbal* can imply a person doesn't have other modes of expressive language or doesn't understand language. But we know that people who don't speak may be able to understand language and may communicate in other ways, like writing, typing, or using a communication device. It's important not to assume that someone who is nonspeaking doesn't have the capacity to understand or use language.

For a term that might be unfamiliar, I provide a definition the first time it appears in the book. If you come across a term and would like its definition, go to the index and find the page where it first appears. For medical terms, I also provide a glossary at the back of the book.

Since many of the children's experiences you'll read about in this book contain confidential medical information, I've altered details to ensure privacy for the children and their families. The details changed for privacy purposes don't alter the relevant facts. All stories represent my collective experience working with thousands of autistic children, adolescents, adults, and their families. In one instance a mother and child requested I use their real names, so I've done so.

Introduction

When I got a late-night message from Kara, the mom of my patient Colin, I thought maybe new concerns had cropped up. Colin was a talented high-school student, cross-country runner, and photographer who'd been my patient since he was two years old. When we met, he'd just been diagnosed with autism, had uncontrolled seizures, and had lost some of his ability to speak. During that time, his parents and I met nearly every week to coordinate his complex medical care and intensive developmental-behavioral therapy program. Together, we found a way through what his parents later called "the storm." Month by month, year by year, with careful attention to his medical care, therapy program, nutrition, sleep, home environment, family relationships, school experiences, and community activities, Colin's health and development improved in remarkable ways. He was doing so well that a full year had passed since we last met, so when Kara sent me a message out of the blue, I read it right away.

Thankfully, things were going well, and Colin was thriving in school and enjoying his extracurricular activities. Kara messaged me because she had read an article that highlighted new findings from autism research studies and was eager to know what the findings meant for Colin. Like so many parents, she wanted to know if the promise of decades of autism research had led to something new that would make a positive difference for her child.

Innovation in autism care is happening at a faster pace today than ever before. Thousands upon thousands of research studies on the biological and behavioral aspects of autism have expanded our knowledge and paved the way for new approaches to care. As a practicing pediatric neurologist, behavior analyst, and autism researcher, I meet parents every day who are urgently curious to know if there's something more they can do for their child's health and development.

The dedication and spirit of these families inspired me to create Cortica, an organization that provides comprehensive autism services spanning medical, developmental, and behavior therapies. Our mission is to offer families a whole-child approach with a single, integrated team that stays up-to-date with the latest cutting-edge research and translates meaningful advances directly to patient care. Ten years ago I started Cortica in a small one-room office in San Diego, California, with a team of three people. The progress we saw in our children and their families was so encouraging that we opened more centers, and today we have twenty-four centers across seven states with a team of more than a thousand doctors and therapists—including pediatric neurologists, pediatricians, psychologists, nurse practitioners, speech-language pathologists, occupational therapists, physical therapists, music therapists, behavior therapists, and mental health professionals—all with expertise in autism and child development and committed to bringing world-class, whole-child care to families across the country and around the world.

Every family seeking autism care deserves a compassionate, integrated team that understands all aspects of whole-child health, but today there simply aren't enough providers to meet the need. Around two million children in the United States—one in thirty-six—have a diagnosis of autism. Research done at Stanford University found that for every autistic child in the United States who receives a needed autism service, eighteen others are waiting. When I speak at conferences or present webinars to parents seeking to learn more about how to help their children, they often ask me how to create a whole-child approach where they live, with the resources available to them. I wrote *Magnificent Minds* as a guide for how to do this.

Wherever you are and whatever services are available to you, the knowledge you'll find in this book can help you create a holistic program to nurture your whole child and support your whole family, so you can all experience more fulfillment and joy.

In this book I share what I believe every parent of an autistic child should know and provide a road map for supporting your child—from medical testing to nutritional and pharmacological interventions to the latest device-based therapies to the most important developmental, behavioral, and mental health strategies. You'll gain a clear understanding of what autism means and how to think about autism's core features and co-occurring conditions. You'll learn how to use this information to understand your child's unique neurodevelopmental profile and to create optimal learning experiences at home, in therapy sessions, in school, and in the community. You'll discover how to support every aspect of your child's health, and since autism doesn't show up the same way in any two people, you'll learn how to make informed decisions based on a deep understanding of your child's unique body and brain. You'll learn how to foster the development of brain networks for sensory, motor, cognitive, language, social, and emotional abilities to further your child along their own unique developmental trajectory, rather than forcing them to fit a neurotypical profile, which can cause lasting harm to mental and emotional health. You'll learn how to recognize and nurture your child's intelligence, abilities, and gifts, and you'll learn to use the principles of neurodiversity to guide the choices you make.

No other child is just like your own, so the children you'll meet in this book may be very different from your own child, or you may see some similarities. Either way, I think you'll find that by looking through these windows into the worlds of other autistic children, you'll learn something new that will expand your thinking and help as you make important decisions for your child. I have also included exercises throughout the book and encourage you to do them as they come up, because the exercises in earlier chapters set you up for later chapters. To make the information and exercises as useful and accessible as possible, read the book with a journal or notepad and a pen or pencil, or with any preferred device you have for taking notes.

For years, I searched for a book that I could recommend to parents—those just beginning to learn about autism as well as those with decades of experience. I looked for a book with all the essential information, the "liquid gold"—something a busy parent could get through while keeping up with the demands of life. I couldn't find that book, so I set out to write it. The information you'll find in these pages draws from thousands of books and articles written by doctors, psychologists, neuroscientists, therapists, and parents, as well as autistic authors. My understanding of autism and the approach of caring for the whole child is based on more than twenty years of clinical practice and informed by my own research, including studies looking at brain networks and brain chemistry in autism, the biological basis and meaning of intelligence, pathways to communication for nonspeaking children, and developmental outcomes made possible by a whole-child approach. This book brings it all together.

My message in this book is directed to parents, but the information is for anyone who wants to create more opportunities for autistic people to experience greater health, well-being, and joy. For professionals who've seen the limitations of our current state of fragmented care, I hope this book provides inspiration to collaborate deeply with professionals from other disciplines, who may see things differently than you do, and to use a whole-child approach to bring cohesion to what may at first appear to be irreconcilable views.

As a teen growing up in Toledo, Ohio, I volunteered as a counselor at a summer camp for children with autism, epilepsy, cerebral palsy, spina bifida, and other neurological differences. The joy and beauty of these children's neurodiversity motivated me to study the science of brain development. Nearly three decades later, my own nephew was diagnosed with autism, and being the aunt to this beloved boy has given me an invaluable personal perspective. In the children at the summer camp in Toledo, in my nephew, and in all the autistic children and adults I've had the privilege to know, I've seen what neurologist Oliver Sacks saw when he first met Temple Grandin—people "full of health, of depth, of deep human strivings."

Through the beautiful days and the inevitable stormy ones, I hope this book will help your child and family find greater connection, meaning, and purpose. Most of all, I hope the knowledge you find in these pages will help you discover your child's true magnificence.

Part 1

WHAT AUTISM MEANS

Chapter 1

SEEING THE WHOLE CHILD

Understanding *All* of Autism

Our ability to influence our circumstances
depends on how we see things.

—Jon Kabat-Zinn, PhD, mindfulness teacher

The hotel lobby was buzzing with parents, doctors, therapists, and educators, all picking up registration packets for the four-day conference. A quick review of the program showed more than sixty presenters covering topics like navigating school-based services, approaches to behavior management, augmentative and alternative communication, strategies for executive functioning, diet and nutrition, gastrointestinal conditions, immune function, and my own talk on seizures. Just the titles and descriptions of the presentations were a lot to take in.

As I rifled through my packet for my presenter's badge, I heard a familiar voice call my name. I turned around to see Joanna, the mom of my young patient Andy, a vibrant three-year-old with brown hair and blue eyes, who had autism, epilepsy, and a genetic condition. In addition to reading everything she could about Andy's diagnoses,

Joanna was caring for Andy's two-month-old brother, so I was amazed that she always arrived for appointments with a list of insightful questions. I was also amazed that she'd managed to make it to the conference on an early Saturday morning.

"Hi, Joanna! What do you think of the conference?" I asked.

Her bright smile faded and tears filled her eyes. She said, "It's too much. I don't know how to do this."

I leaned forward and put a hand on her arm. "Just take in what you can and that's more than enough. Write down your questions, and we'll go through them the next time we meet." She nodded and we walked through the crowded hall together.

Unfortunately, being overwhelmed by information about autism is common. Just twenty years ago, information was hard to find, but now there's more than any parent or professional can possibly absorb. The sheer volume can lead parents on an endless search fueled by the belief "If I knew more and did more, my child would be better off." Many parents I meet have tried dozens, sometimes hundreds, of interventions. Even after pouring significant personal and financial resources into therapies, they doubt whether they've done enough. That persistent uncertainty takes a powerful toll. It can make you feel as if your efforts have been a failure when the truth is that they've been heroic. If you find yourself fluctuating between wanting to do more and not knowing if you can handle more, you're not alone.

Having a full understanding of autism doesn't mean knowing every elimination diet, nutritional supplement, medication, or developmental-behavioral approach ever developed. Having a full understanding means having a holistic framework to build a program that supports all aspects of health and behavior that are important for your child, based on their unique profile. It means knowing where new pieces of information fit and what to do with them, and it means becoming aware of all the people and places that can help your child flourish. With this understanding, you'll know you're doing the best for your child.

Autism Plus (+)

Autism is a single word, but not a single thing. Each autistic person is a unique individual with autistic characteristics that are unique, and each person may also have a unique set of *co-occurring features* (the *plus* in *autism plus*).

Today there is a mountain of information about autism. Researchers, doctors, therapists, public health officials, product manufacturers, service providers, advocacy organizations, parents, and autistic people themselves have strong views. As you might expect, they don't all agree on what autism is or how it should be approached. But they *do* agree that autism is multidimensional. As you begin to see a fuller picture of your child, you'll recognize that these dimensions aren't so much problems that need to be managed or fixed as they are opportunities to better understand and nurture your child and their magnificent mind.

AUTISTIC CHARACTERISTICS

Autistic characteristics are *human* characteristics that should be viewed as variations along a continuum of human traits, not as deficits or deficiencies. These characteristics fall into two categories:

(1) Differences in social communication and interaction, such as
- a toddler who has no trouble hearing but doesn't respond when their name is called

- a five-year-old who shows signs of enjoying toys and other activities but doesn't share that enjoyment with others (doesn't look at others or include others)
- an eight-year-old who can talk at length about favorite topics but doesn't engage in back-and-forth conversation
- a teenager or an adult who's unsure what others are thinking or feeling and may cope by avoiding social situations

(2) Differences in flexibility with thoughts, behaviors, activities, or sensory responses to the environment, such as
- a toddler who lines up toys rather than playing with them in other ways
- a four-year-old who frequently flips light switches on and off
- a seven-year-old who seeks out certain sensations (such as certain smells or textures) but who covers their ears to avoid certain sounds
- a ten-year-old who likes to arrange objects in a specific way and doesn't respond well to small changes in daily routines
- a teenager or an adult who has a specific topic of intense focus that occupies much of their time, thought, and conversation with others

These are just some examples of autism's core characteristics. It's important to remember that autistic differences in social interaction and behavioral flexibility are unique to each person. No two people are the same, and characteristics can change quite a bit over time, so the autistic characteristics your child has today are likely to change as your child grows and develops.

Autistic characteristics also seem to differ between males and females. Some research studies have found autistic girls and women are more likely to

- recognize when social interactions are expected
- imitate others in social interactions
- be described by others as "passive" or "shy"
- show characteristics of perfectionism
- have higher language abilities
- have intense interests that involve people or animals rather than items or objects

What are your child's autistic characteristics? If your child has had an autism diagnostic evaluation, the results of that evaluation probably included a detailed description of these characteristics. But rather than relying on a professional's observations, try to focus on what you've noticed about your child.

Write down your own observations about

- how your child communicates with others
- how your child acts around others, including other children, adults, family members, and strangers
- how your child responds when other people approach them
- what your child prefers to do during free time
- how your child responds to sensory information from the environment, like what they see, hear, smell, taste, or touch

Some of the things you've written down are likely to be features of autism, but others may not be. From my perspective, the distinction doesn't matter all that much. What's more important is that you're noticing your child's characteristics and that your overall understanding of your child is growing. Throughout this book I share information and exercises to help you do this because the knowledge you have of your child will empower you to support their development in exciting new directions.

CO-OCCURRING FEATURES

Anything that isn't captured in the two core categories of autistic features but that happens more frequently in autistic than in non-autistic people is considered a *co-occurring feature* of autism. Co-occurring features include a range of medical, developmental, behavioral, and mental health features.

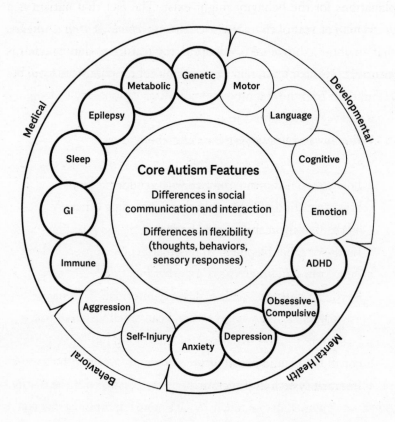

Research in this area has blossomed in recent years. For some people these are simply characteristics that shape their personality. Others, who meet the threshold for a medical diagnosis, can benefit from medical care. About 90 percent of autistic children have at least one co-occurring condition, and more than half will experience four or more co-occurring conditions. Unfortunately, these conditions aren't always recognized, so they're often unaddressed. A child's self-injurious behavior, for example, might be called "part of autism" without anyone looking deeper to see if gastrointestinal pain, headache, heightened stress, sensory processing differences, or other explanations for the behavior might exist. The fact that autism is a *description* of a set of characteristics and *not a biological cause* means that attributing any core or co-occurring feature to autism itself is incorrect. This common mistake prevents appropriate steps from being taken to find the true underlying reasons.

Co-occurring medical symptoms or conditions:
- Genetic conditions (these conditions are due to alterations in genes, chromosomes, or other genetic information)
- Mitochondrial and other metabolic disorders (these conditions affect the way the body converts nutrients into energy or other biochemical processes)
- Epilepsy (seizures)
- Sleep disturbances (such as difficulty falling asleep or staying asleep)
- Gastrointestinal (GI) symptoms (such as abdominal pain, constipation, and heartburn)
- Immune system dysfunction

Co-occurring developmental, behavioral, or mental health symptoms or conditions:
- Delays or other differences in motor, language, cognitive, or emotional development

- Attention-deficit hyperactivity disorder (ADHD)
- Obsessive-compulsive disorder
- Depression
- Anxiety
- Self-injury
- Aggression

Research studies have found that some of these features tend to accompany each other. For example, epilepsy and sleep disturbance often occur together. This could be because both can be caused by differences in how neurons (nerve cells) connect with each other. Some studies have found that GI symptoms and sleep disturbance also frequently occur together, and this may be because GI symptoms like heartburn, constipation, and abdominal pain can cause discomfort that keeps a child from falling asleep or wakes a child from sleep. Children with an underlying genetic condition are also more likely to have epilepsy and cognitive disability. So far, research studies have not consistently shown differences in co-occurring medical conditions between boys and girls.

A Holistic Framework

Many researchers dedicate their entire career to studying just one of the core characteristics or co-occurring features of autism, but for parents, the path to building an effective program for your child begins by adopting a much wider view.

The approach I take is to imagine the inside of a cell in the brain called a neuron. Your child's brain has close to a hundred billion neurons.

Neuron

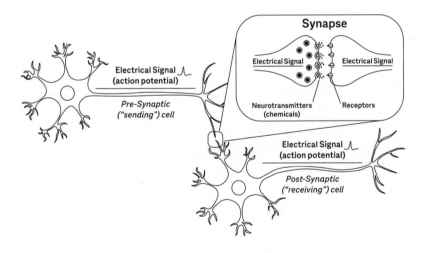

Neurons have electrical and chemical functions. Electrical signals travel within neurons, and chemical transmission happens in the spaces between neurons, called synapses.

Synapse

Electrical Signal (action potential)

Pre-Synaptic ("sending") cell

Electrical Signal

Neurotransmitters (chemicals)

Electrical Signal

Receptors

Electrical Signal (action potential)

Post-Synaptic ("receiving") cell

How neurons work at a chemical and electrical level is different for different children. In part 2 of this book, you'll learn ways to understand more about your child's brain chemistry and electrical activity.

Zooming out to a slightly larger view, we can consider how your child's neurons communicate with one another to create brain networks in each of these major developmental domains:

- Sensory (how we sense the world around us)
- Motor (how we move our bodies)
- Cognitive (how we think, including attention, memory, planning, and problem-solving)
- Language (how we understand and use words to communicate)
- Social (how we interact with other people)
- Emotional (how we process feelings)

These are the fundamental brain networks for child development that you'll learn more about in part 2.

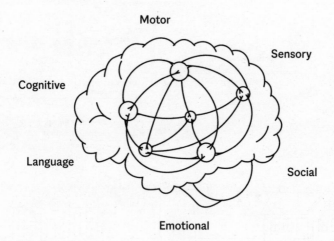

Zooming out further, we look at the rest of your child's body to consider the function of gastrointestinal, immune, and other body systems, which all influence your child's brain development.

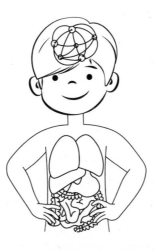

Finally, we can step back for an even broader view, to see your whole child and how their growth—represented in this image by the tree—is influenced by the people and settings around them at home, in school, and in the wider community.

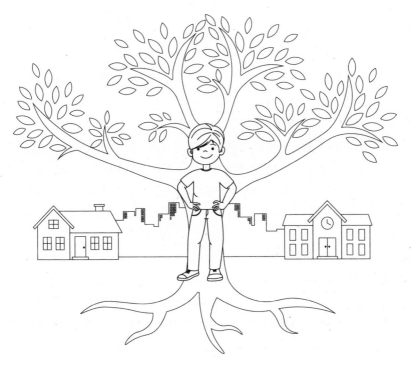

This approach to viewing autism, in which we can zoom in to a microscopic level and zoom out to a child's place in their home, school, and community, allows us to appreciate how everything is connected. Though the core characteristics of autism relate to the biggest-picture view—how a person experiences and engages with the world around them—underneath are multiple layers of brain and body function that each offer an opportunity for investigation, understanding, and individualized support. Seeing the whole interconnected view allows you to support your child in the most important ways. Tunnel vision, on the other hand, can make the path forward more difficult because the full benefit of any particular intervention can't be realized when other areas are unsupported. Without a balanced, holistic approach, interventions intended to help are more likely to cause harm.

Some common examples of tunnel vision in autism care include

- lack of carry-through with tests or treatments for co-occurring medical conditions
- hyperfocus on diet and nutritional supplementation but lack of follow-through with home activities recommended by a child's therapists
- seeking more hours of behavior therapy, also called applied behavior analysis (ABA), than recommended by the therapy team while not following through with recommended sensory-motor therapies (e.g., occupational, physical, and/or music therapy) or recommended medical tests and therapies
- overmedication for behaviors that could be effectively addressed through changes to the daily routine and home environment

In a whole-child approach to autism, you can visualize your child's development in this way:

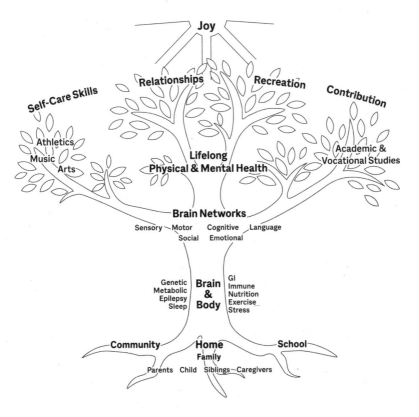

I use this framework to help the parents and professionals I work with see how the elements of whole-child autism care come together. Starting from the bottom, we see that supporting the health of the home and well-being of all family members, including parents, child, siblings, and other caregivers, builds strong roots for child development. Improving a child's experiences and learning opportunities at school and in the wider community also contributes to a stable foundation for growth.

The trunk of the tree represents the health of the brain and body, which includes a thorough understanding of and appropriate support based on your child's genetic and metabolic profile and any co-occurring medical conditions. It also includes supporting your child's nutrition, exercise, and stress reduction—all of which make a positive difference for your child's development.

On that foundation of health, the tree grows branches, which represent brain networks across all major developmental domains: sensory, motor, cognitive, language, social, and emotional.

The tree then extends into higher-level skills in athletics, music, and arts and in academic and vocational studies.

Optimizing physical and mental health is a lifelong goal and supports your child's success in self-care skills, relationships, recreation, and making a contribution to the world.

Finally, the experience of joy, like the rays of the sun, is what nourishes success in each of the other areas. At the same time, the reason for supporting all the other areas is to enable the experience of joy. Keeping this top of mind will guide you well in the decisions you make for each step of your child's care.

Your Child's Unique Profile

To understand your child's unique profile, use the holistic framework to help organize your knowledge. If you're not ready to answer these questions, don't worry. Part 2 of this book will guide you step-by-step to understand each part of your child's unique profile.

Home and Family
Who lives at home with your child?
How are they doing (physical and mental health)?
What support do they have?
How are relationships at home?
How does it feel at home (e.g., safe, comfortable, peaceful,
    stressful, chaotic, unpredictable, etc.)?

Community

What does your child do in the community (e.g., activities, outings, etc.)?

What are these experiences like for your child and your family?

School

What is your child's school setting?

What experiences—academic, social, and others—does your child have at school? (consider both positive and negative experiences)

How does your child feel at school?

Brain and Body

What do you know about your child's health in each of these areas?

Genetic

Metabolic

Seizure

Sleep

Gastrointestinal (GI)

Immune

Nutrition

Exercise

Stress

Brain Networks

What do you know about your child in each of these developmental domains?

Sensory

Motor

Cognitive

Language

Social

Emotional

Lifelong Physical and Mental Health

What are some things you're doing to support your child's physical and mental health?

Athletics, Music, and Arts

What experiences does your child have with athletics, music, and arts?

Academic and Vocational Studies

What are your child's experiences in academic and vocational studies?

How do you think these could expand in the future?

Self-Care Skills

What self-care skills does your child have?

What's being done to support and grow these skills?

Relationships

What are the important relationships in your child's life?

How are these relationships supported?

How could these grow in the future?

Recreation

What recreational experiences does your child have?

How could more opportunities be created?

Contribution

Every person has a contribution to make to the world. It can look many different ways. Making a contribution creates a sense of purpose.

What is your child's contribution?
What could it be in the future?

Joy

What brings your child joy?
How does your child bring you joy?

The many dimensions of autism—the core characteristics and the co-occurring features—along with each element of the child development tree create a *neurodevelopmental* profile that's one-of-a-kind. No two profiles are the same. This is what autistic author and professor Dr. Stephen Shore means when he says, "If you've met one person with autism, you've met one person with autism." Knowing this, you can see that the way forward becomes more about understanding and supporting your child so that they flourish along their unique developmental path, instead of imposing a set of requirements or goals based on typical developmental milestones.

> *There is no one way to be autistic. Some autistic people can speak, and some autistic people need to communicate in other ways. . . . Some autistic people need a lot of help in their day-to-day lives, and some autistic people only need a little help. . . . All of us experience autism differently, but we all contribute to the world in meaningful ways. We all deserve understanding and acceptance.*
>
> —AUTISTIC SELF ADVOCACY NETWORK

Seeing That Your Child Is Whole

Choosing a holistic view means seeing your child through a lens of possibilities rather than limitations and by abilities rather than deficits. It means identifying areas where your child would benefit from support, while always keeping in view how everything fits together and how everything is connected.

It's possible that past experiences and the messages you've received from other people may make it hard for you to do this. Maybe you've been at a school meeting, medical appointment, or developmental evaluation where others described your child in a way that felt off, like they didn't truly see your child. This happens because, sadly, professionals are still taught to define children by limitations. Professionals in the field of child development spend years learning language, concepts, and practices that splinter and fragment, rather than integrate and unify. Even the most well-meaning professionals can struggle to replace a deficit-oriented, compartmentalized approach with one that's more holistic and life-affirming. Interacting with professionals who unwittingly impose these negative views can be a traumatic experience.

It's important to avoid seeing your child through a lens of limitations rather than one of possibilities, by deficits rather than abilities, or as anything less than whole. This isn't accurate or helpful, and ultimately does great harm. If you and the other people most important in your child's life adopt this view, your child will, too. Once your child internalizes this view as truth, the opportunity to fulfill their actual potential becomes vanishingly small.

Understanding all of autism means knowing that no matter what developmental skills are not yet reached or what behavior needs to be addressed, your child is already whole and complete, just as they are.

Here are some things that parents who adopt a holistic view have told me about their children:

"He still gets tired easily. When he's tired, he's clumsier, and his speech is less clear. But he's really starting to bond with his brother. He looks for him and asks him to play, which he never used to do. He got a part in his school play, and he loves it. He really comes alive on stage."

—MOM OF NOAH, EIGHT-YEAR-OLD WITH AUTISM,
GENETIC SYNDROME, AND MITOCHONDRIAL DYSFUNCTION

"Her teacher at school changed last month, and since then she won't get on the bus. We're going to observe her class next Monday. She started biting her hands again. I think we need to restart her medication while we sort out what's happening at school. With her music therapist, she started writing songs, and last week she watched The Wizard of Oz *from start to finish. She's never watched a full movie before. She really loves music."*

—DAD OF EMI, TEN-YEAR-OLD WITH AUTISM
AND SELF-INJURY WHO IS NONSPEAKING

"His seizures went up last month. Sometimes he gets out of control and starts throwing things. His dad has to hold him for a few minutes until he calms down. But we're seeing him be more aware and engaged at school and at home. He really seems happy, and his personality is showing through. He's sleeping better than ever before."

—MOM OF ZAC, EIGHTEEN-YEAR-OLD WITH AUTISM,
EPILEPSY, AND AGGRESSIVE BEHAVIOR

"She's still not able to say more than a few words, and she's only eating a few foods. But she's been swimming three or four times a

week, and she's such a strong swimmer. Her freestyle is really good and she's learning backstroke."

—DAD OF SARA, FOUR-YEAR-OLD WITH AUTISM
AND SPEECH-LANGUAGE DELAY

"The hardest part for him is still being able to focus. He needs a lot of reminders and someone with him to help him finish whatever activity he's supposed to be doing. But for the first time we were able to go on a family trip last month. We never thought it would be possible. We went to Italy and France. It was life-changing for all of us."

—MOM OF ARJUN, TWENTY-YEAR-OLD WITH AUTISM AND ADHD

"She hasn't made a lot of progress with her speech. She's able to say some phrases, but it's not fluent. One day I saw her watching videos on YouTube about stars and planets, so I signed her up for an online astronomy camp. She sat through every lecture. I couldn't believe it! She can't tell us yet, but I know there's a lot she's thinking about."

—MOM OF GINA, TWELVE-YEAR-OLD WITH AUTISM AND EPILEPSY

Adopting a holistic view doesn't happen overnight. It happens by learning to think about things differently and replacing old ideas with new ones. As you'll see in the next chapter, the ideas that are part of the neurodiversity movement are among the most important for helping you embrace a holistic view of autism.

Chapter 2

DIFFERENT, NOT LESS

Embracing Neurodiversity

Neurodiversity refers ... to the limitless
variability of human cognition and
the uniqueness of each human mind.

—Judy Singer, sociologist

In the book *Different . . . Not Less*, the brilliant autistic author and
scientist Dr. Temple Grandin shares inspiring stories of people with
autism and ADHD. Through these stories—from veterinary surgeon
Neil to dancer Leonora to tour guide and history buff Charli to inves-
tor and philanthropist Richard—we see the value of minds that think
differently. Grandin herself is a professor of animal sciences, a prolific
author, and an outspoken proponent of autism rights who has made
Time magazine's list of the hundred most influential people in the
world.

As you embark on the next steps of the whole-child path, I hope
you'll remember these stories and seek out others. You have a distinct
role in helping your child understand their unique differences and

finding ways they can explore and discover their own gifts. No one can do this better than you. When you see your child's characteristics as potential gifts and opportunities, you open the door for them and for everyone who knows them to do the same. And that's when all people can start to understand the profound truth that autistic people are different, not less.

The Biology of Neurodiversity

There are countless ways that one brain differs from another. *Neurodiversity*—a word that comes from *neurological* and *diversity*—describes the natural differences in how people think, learn, and behave. Thousands of genes influence how our brains work, and these genes come in different versions called *variants*. People have different combinations of variants that together help create what we might think of as a unique neurological fingerprint. These neurological differences are an important reason why people experience and engage with the world in different ways.

For example, a gene that's received a lot of attention from neuroscientists is one called *brain-derived neurotrophic factor* (BDNF). BDNF helps the brain grow new connections and supports learning and memory. A unique feature of BDNF is that levels of BDNF protein in your body can increase when you exercise, and this is one of the reasons why exercising can help you improve your thinking, memory, and mood. How much BDNF your body makes from exercise is related to which gene variant you have, and there are tests that can determine this. Researchers have also found that a person's BDNF variant influences how likely they are to have learning disabilities, anxiety, depression, and conditions like Alzheimer's and Parkinson's.

BDNF is just one example of thousands of genes that influence brain function.

So the genes we're born with make each of us unique. But our individuality doesn't stop there. The life experiences we have also change our brain. Neuroscientists call this *experience-driven neuroplasticity*. Brain networks are like muscles in the sense that when we use them, they get stronger and grow. That's why musicians who spend much of their time listening to and making music have enlargement in the parts of their brain that process sound and the parts that plan and carry out intricate movements. Any specific skill that we practice for long periods of time can stimulate change in the brain. For example, people who regularly practice meditation show differences in brain electrical activity from people who don't.

So genes, experiences, and other factors come together and cause differences in the brain's physical characteristics, neurochemistry, and electrical activity. The size and shape of your brain, the structures inside, the architecture of brain pathways, and the balance and activity of neurochemicals are genuinely unique. You are not only different from every other person who's alive now; you're also different from everyone who's ever been alive or ever will be. No two brains are the same! When we understand the nature of neurodiversity, we see that there's no single "right" or "normal" way of thinking, learning, or behaving. We also see that neurological differences between people shouldn't be viewed as deficits, shortcomings, or failures.

The Rise of a Human Rights Movement

Neurodiversity is rooted in biology, but its significance goes far beyond the brain and body into the realm of human rights. Steve Silberman, author of the *New York Times* bestseller *NeuroTribes*, describes neurodiversity as "the rallying cry of the first new civil rights movement to take off in the twenty-first century." The neurodiversity movement is about social justice for "neurological minorities" (or neurominorities). Just as the long history of injustice toward racial minorities in the United States led to the birth of the civil rights movement of the 1960s, the history of inequality toward people with neurological differences has given rise to the neurodiversity movement.

Neurodiversity refers to

- the neurological differences among people that lead to differences in how we experience and engage with the world around us
- the viewpoint that these differences in neurology and behavior aren't deficits or deviations—that there's no single right way of being
- the human rights movement that has emerged in the twenty-first century to champion these ideas and enact changes in our society and our culture

The neurodiversity movement grew out of the broader disability rights movement that started in the United States in the 1960s. The disability rights movement made us aware of the way societies create the experience of disability through barriers, negative attitudes, and exclusionary practices. The values of a society and culture determine the meaning and consequences of a person's physical or mental characteristics. Ideas about which ways of thinking, communicating, and behaving are preferred, and which ways are outside the bounds of "normal," are created by people. They aren't somehow predetermined. As Dr. Thomas Armstrong, author of *The Power of Neurodiversity*,

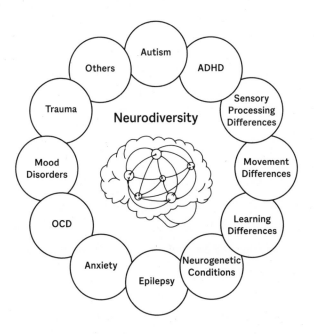

says, "Whether you are regarded as disabled or gifted depends largely on when and where you were born. . . . No brain exists in a social vacuum."

People with disabilities experience stigma, meaning they bear the negative attitudes and discriminatory practices that go along with being seen as less. This happens when a characteristic is viewed as being different from an expected "normal" identity—whether it's a physical feature, health condition, or trait related to gender, sexuality, or race. These attitudes and practices stem from the mistaken belief that there's a single "normal" way of being, and they're the root cause of tremendous harm. As sociologist Erving Goffman says, stigma disqualifies an individual from full social acceptance and labels an individual as not fully human—not whole. Ideas about what's "normal" can be so ingrained and so widely accepted in a society that they become hard to see.

The disability rights movement also led to the creation of a new word, *ableism*, which has helped bring greater attention to the stigma and inequity that exist toward disabled people. *Ableism* refers to the discrimination and social prejudice against people with disabilities based on the myth that typical abilities are superior. Understanding the pervasive nature of ableism and its many forms is the first step to counteracting these harmful ideas and seeing neurodivergent people as whole and fully human. In recent years, this shift in mindset has been beautifully reflected in books like *Uniquely Human: A Different Way of Seeing Autism*, by speech-language pathologist Barry Prizant, and *How to Be Human: An Autistic Man's Guide to Life*, by autistic Rhodes scholar Jory Fleming.

In recent years, autistic people have also pushed the neurodiversity movement forward by openly identifying as autistic, supporting others to be open and comfortable with this identity, and committing to taking action that supports equal rights for people of all abilities. Their efforts also involve adopting identity-centered language—for example, to be called *autistic* rather than a *person with autism*. Identity-centered (or identity-first) language reflects the growing preference among autistic people to openly identify as autistic. This represents a shift away from person-first language (e.g., *child with autism* or *person with autism*), which can imply that autism is a disorder that someone "has" rather than a valued part of one's identity. Some parents have told me that it can be uncomfortable at first to use identity-centered language for their child, but understanding what it means as part of the neurodiversity movement allows them to embrace it.

What It Means to Be Neurodivergent or Neurodiverse

The neurodiversity movement has introduced new words like *neurodivergent* and *neurodiverse* that signify an important change in how we view neurological differences. *Neurodivergent* describes individuals who have ways of learning, thinking, or behaving that aren't considered typical. *Neurodiverse* describes groups of individuals with various neurological characteristics (i.e., groups that are neurologically diverse). For example, a classroom with students who are neurotypical and students who have neurological differences, such as autism, ADHD, and dyslexia, could be described as a neurodiverse class. Because *neurodiversity*, in its broadest sense, refers to the neurological differences that exist among all people, any group of people could potentially be called neurodiverse, but the term is usually used for groups that include neurological minorities.

The words used to describe neurological differences have historically come from the medical field. Now, for the first time, a civil rights movement has brought new language for talking about these differences. These new words are powerful because they carry with them the principles of the neurodiversity movement. When we use these terms with our children, family members, professionals, and others in the broader community, we help to promote the goals of the neurodiversity movement.

Debates in
the Neurodiversity Movement

A key debate in the neurodiversity movement is whether neurological differences should be considered primarily positive (traits that should be celebrated and not changed) or primarily negative (symptoms of illness that should be eliminated or cured if possible). There's no easy answer. This is partly because of the vast spectrum of neurological differences but also because the question is best answered by each neurodivergent person for themselves. Of the many voices that have taken part in this debate, John Elder Robison strikes a balance. He advocates for the view that neurological differences can produce both disabilities and strengths. He expresses the need to value neurological differences *and* provide appropriate supports, services, and accommodations. As Temple Grandin says, autism is both a disability and a gift.

Another question being debated is how health-care services might change for people with neurological differences if they aren't viewed as deficits. It's important to recognize that a shift from seeing autistic traits as deficits to differences doesn't mean health-care services should become scarcer. In fact, improved access to quality health care is essential for achieving equity and inclusion for neurodivergent people. Inferior-quality health care and poor access to health care are well-known forms of institutionalized discrimination. Unfortunately, many neurodivergent people experience inequity in the form of inadequate services for neurodevelopment in many parts of our country and around the world. Services are fragmented, which diminishes access and quality, and health-care professionals often lack neurodiversity training, so families continue to suffer from encounters in health-care settings where a deficit-oriented view of autism and other neurological differences is still ingrained. But fortunately, the rise of "neurodiversity-affirming intervention" is helping to change this.

The essential components of neurodiversity-affirming intervention are

- supporting a person's development while not attempting to change personal characteristics unless those characteristics cause harm or discomfort to the individual or infringe on others' rights
- addressing, whenever possible, any external factors in the environment that get in the way of a person feeling included and accepted or that reduce a person's opportunities for enjoyment, learning, and advancement
- acknowledging the strengths, preferences, and values of a person and making a concerted effort to understand what these are and how they change over time
- using language that shows respect for people with all forms of neurological differences and avoiding language that suggests deficiency

You Can Make a Difference

Every citizen, organization, and nation has an important role to play in the neurodiversity movement, including you, your child, and your family. There are many ways you can help your child and everyone who interacts with them to understand and embrace the principles of neurodiversity.

A great first step is to find space in your own life for the practices described earlier that are part of neurodiversity-affirming intervention.

- Make a list of your child's strengths and preferences.
- Try, if you can, to learn about their values: what's important to your child and why.
- Use language that shows respect and try not to change your child's characteristics unless they're causing harm or discomfort to them or causing harm to others.
- Whenever you can, try to adapt the environment to reduce your child's exposure to negative experiences, but also look for opportunities to expand their horizons in ways that don't overwhelm them.
- Let family members, teachers, therapists, and others in your child's life know what you're doing and why, and tell them how they can help.

Nothing makes me happier than when parents come to my office and tell me about something they did to recognize and support their child's unique gifts. One mother made a presentation for her son's teachers and other school staff, with photos showing him skiing, running a 5K race, mountain biking, and eating at his favorite restaurant. She told me she wanted to help them see more of who her son is and not make assumptions about him because he doesn't speak. Other parents I work with give out copies of stories, articles, or books that they want other parents or professionals to learn from. I've received many of these and appreciate them every time. No one has taught me more than the families I work with.

One parent who used social media to educate the world about neurodiversity is an inventor and engineer known for his creative and engaging approach to teaching science. In a YouTube video that's been viewed more than thirty-four million times, Mark Rober shares the story of his autistic son. He describes his son's unique gifts as perseverance, bringing happiness to others, finding simple joys, laughter, and bringing out positive qualities in others such as patience and compassion.

Neurodiversity is, above all, about recognizing that every human being brings unique gifts to the world. Many of the ideas around neurodiversity, its biological basis, and its social and political significance can be complex, but we can make them understandable and accessible to people of different ages, backgrounds, and abilities. Every action you take to support the neurodiversity movement makes a real difference to your child and to the world.

Chapter 3

WHAT'S STRONG WITH ME?

Strengths Outweigh Weaknesses

Our differences are our strengths.

—Mickey Rowe, autistic actor

The question "What's strong with me?" startled me the first time I heard it. Because we direct so many of our day-to-day thoughts to what's wrong, it can feel odd to ask what's strong. But this simple question has the power to release the tight hold that problems have on our thoughts and open a new way of thinking.

We've all had moments when problems seem so big that it's hard to think of anything else. Those are exactly the times when bringing strengths to the forefront matters most. Mindfulness teacher Jon Kabat-Zinn reminds us, "As long as you are breathing, there is more right with you than wrong, no matter what is wrong."

Many parents I work with embrace this idea. They focus on their child's strengths and make sure others do, too. But some parents, when told their child's strengths, respond by saying, "Yes, but . . ." They redirect the focus back to what's wrong. I believe the goal is to strike a balance—to get to "Yes, *and* . . ." Of course, we should take every action to understand and attend to autism and its co-occurring features, but none of that matters if we don't highlight and grow your child's strengths.

What's a Strength?

I think of a strength as something someone can do, and when they do it, it serves them well. A strength is an ability. Everyone has strengths.

But not all people think about strengths this way. People often mistake strengths as abilities that are defined by comparison with others' abilities or with some external standard. Some researchers even define strengths as only those skills that are executed nearly perfectly every time. By that standard, only machines and super-heroes have strengths. It's no wonder we have a hard time recognizing strengths in our children and ourselves.

Defining strengths by comparison doesn't make sense. Consider, for example, something you do that serves you well. Maybe it's jog-ging, hiking, swimming, cooking, organizing, following a schedule, making people laugh, showing people you care, helping others learn, or any of the skills that help you to be the kind of parent, friend, citizen, and person that you want to be. I consider my capacity for mindfulness and meditation a strength, but if I compared myself with a Zen master, it would probably look more like a weakness. Some people might argue that the comparison should be with the "norm" or "average" level of ability. In that case, would a skill need to be better than half the people in the world to be a strength? It's impossible to know how we compare with so many others. And even if we could know, it wouldn't mean very much. A person's skill in any area and how it serves them doesn't have much to do with anyone else. The same holds true for all abilities. Sure, we show great admiration for Olympians, world-record holders, and others who demonstrate unique abilities. But those outstanding achievements aren't more important than recognizing and growing individual strengths to advance toward personal goals and maximize potential.

So strengths can't be defined through comparison with others, and they can't be defined solely *by* others, including people who are considered experts in child development. It's up to each person— with the support of those closest to them who know them best—to define their own strengths.

Take a moment to complete this strengths-finding exercise about your child. When you're describing a particular event, include what you remember about the setting, what your child was doing, and what others were doing.

Describe some situations when you've seen your child at their best.

Describe times when your child enjoyed interactions with other people.

Describe times when you saw your child overcome a challenge.

Describe some of the ways your child can care for themselves.

Describe how your child expresses joy. (How does your child look when they're happy?)

Describe a time when your child completed a new activity or showed a new ability.

To succeed in this world, we all need to recognize our own strengths. Unfortunately, learning to recognize one's own strengths isn't usually included in individualized education programs or behavior therapy plans, even though it should be. All learning requires a willingness to take risks, and taking risks requires confidence and trust in one's abilities. Your child has a greater chance of achieving their goals if the voice in their head is asking "What's strong with me?" rather than "What's wrong with me?" In the long run, this can also protect against depression, anxiety, and other mental health symptoms. You can shape your child's inner voice and help your child to be led by what they *can* do, not by what they can't.

Negativity Bias

If you did the strengths-finding exercise, then you're well on your way to thinking in terms of strengths instead of deficits. You're already moving away from what psychologists call *negativity bias*, which is a term that refers to the way negative thoughts, emotions, and experiences leave a stronger impression on people than positive or neutral ones. People spend more time and energy thinking about the negative than the positive and tend to view situations as worse than they are. Negative images and words are like magnets. They attract more of our attention. Rick Hanson, psychologist and author of *Hardwiring Happiness*, describes the brain as Velcro for what's bad and Teflon for what's good. When something happens that could be dangerous or threatening, the information travels quickly through the brain to trigger the body's fight-or-flight response, which causes levels of stress hormones like adrenaline and cortisol to rise. Positive experiences, on the other hand, generally don't trigger the same intense response in the brain and body.

Despite the good intentions of professionals, many of them are under the strong influence of negativity bias. So it's not surprising if you've found that the evaluation process for autism has left you, your child, and others who care about your child in a fog of negativity that's hard to see through. In the wise words of autistic author Tito Mukhopadhyay, "People love to take special interests in the 'cannots' and not the 'cans.'" The language that physicians, psychologists, and therapists have for describing problems is extensive. From the earliest stages of training, we are taught to shine a light on deficits, and we spend years—sometimes decades—learning how to do that with precision. In my role as a pediatric neurologist my job is to gather information on a child's health and development and determine the appropriate medical diagnoses. In the medical record this is called a problem list. Sometimes the list is quite long, like this one for a six-year-old boy I saw recently in my office:

- Autism spectrum disorder
- Attention deficit hyperactivity disorder
- Mixed receptive-expressive language disorder
- Developmental coordination disorder
- Sleep disorder
- Chronic constipation
- Feeding disorder
- Hypotonia (low muscle tone)

In my early medical training as a student and resident, I felt a sense of accomplishment each time I arrived at a set of diagnoses for a patient. Now, twenty years later, it gives me a knot in my stomach. Of course, I know why it's necessary. The labels give a child access to essential medical tests, therapy services, and other resources that can be life-changing. Our institutions and systems are set up this way. Because of that, I have to define a child by disorders, deficits, and symptoms in order to give them access to the supports and resources they deserve. I try to prepare parents beforehand to minimize the negative impact these labels might have. I tell them that their extra-ordinary child with a bright future isn't changed by the medical terms. In fact, the future is brighter now because we know what we should do. But I also feel that whatever I say, it's not always enough to offset the effects of seeing their child defined by deficits and disorders, de-scribed by a list of problems.

Advances in integrative health and functional medicine are gradu-ally opening new doors to health and wellness that rely less on the conventional deficit-based model. These newer approaches recognize the importance of nutrition, lifestyle, and emotional well-being for re-storing health. They apply state-of-the-art techniques to investigate and treat the physiological processes that negatively impact health while using a person-centered approach instead of a disease-centered ap-proach. This model has been slower to make its way to pediatrics, but efforts to establish curricula, training, and certification programs for pediatric integrative health and functional medicine are growing. Per-haps most exciting are the benefits being seen in chronic neurological, psychiatric, autoimmune, and other conditions in children and adults, where the effectiveness of conventional medicine has been limited.

Even before my patient Michelle was born, her parents knew they wanted to take an integrative approach to her health because that's the approach they took for their own health. They focused on nutri-tion, an active lifestyle, and prioritizing emotional well-being. So when Michelle began to show developmental delays at one year of age, their search for a physician who could support her neurological needs and their desire for an integrative health approach led them to me. When Michelle's genetic testing revealed a diagnosis of Rett syn-drome, her parents understood that intensive medical interventions would be needed. Michelle would likely develop seizures and would need regular medical tests to monitor the health of her heart, gastro-intestinal tract, and bones. She would also probably need multiple medications and medical procedures. They understood and were committed to doing it all. But they also wanted all the elements of a holistic, integrative approach. They were concerned that the Rett syndrome diagnosis might rule out an integrated approach for Michelle. I was happy to assure them that a holistic approach was even *more* important for her because she needed many components of care. The more complex a child's needs are, the more important it is to have a person-centered view, to recognize and nurture strengths, and to focus on emotional well-being for the child and all family members.

Choices you make today can create a more balanced, holistic, and invigorating path for your child. Try to begin each day, each activity, each conversation by leading with strengths instead of problems. The problems will always make themselves known. As we know, they're magnets for attention. But you can choose to replace a problem-centered view with a strengths-based view and put problems in their place.

Putting Problems in Their Place

Problems have a way of taking over our thoughts and emotions. The idea that problems deserve to be put in their place comes from an approach to psychotherapy called narrative therapy (or narrative practices). Developed in the 1980s by therapists Michael White and David Epston, this approach recognizes that we all have a life story—a way that we understand and weave together the events of our lives. This story, or narrative, links together experiences and gives them meaning to help us make sense of our lives. Problems usually dominate these stories and cause a great deal of distress. In narrative therapy, the primary source of distress is the problem-saturated life story, not something unchangeable within the person. Once we see that we construct problems from a set of ideas and expectations, we can deconstruct and even reconstruct them. We do this by recognizing that the problem is separate from the person: the problem is the problem; the person is not the problem.

Many autistic characteristics have been framed as problems, but when we look at them more closely, we see that they have purpose and meaningful benefits. Repetitive movements known as stereotypies, for example, can help a child regulate their emotional state and can help them process information from the environment. Reduced eye contact can help someone manage the information they're receiving about other people and in this way reduce visual input that may be overstimulating. Echolalia, the repetition of words just spoken by another person, can help a person process language they've just heard and engage the systems involved in speech. A strong interest in a topic or activity that's thought to be restricting or limiting can be understood instead as a passion that should be nurtured and expanded.

Building a Strengths-Based Approach

More and more people are recognizing the benefits of a strengths-based approach in fields ranging from education to health care to business. People across all ages and abilities do better when we put our efforts toward building on their strengths.

In autism services a strengths-based approach means creating the best possible *person-environment fit*. This means adapting the environment to suit a child's developmental profile and adding supports to help a child to successfully navigate the learning environment.

Important elements of your child's developmental profile include

- sensory characteristics: how your child processes different types of sensory information
- motor qualities: how your child moves within an environment
- cognitive abilities: like how your child thinks, focuses, remembers, and reasons
- communication abilities: how your child understands others and expresses himself or herself
- social-emotional characteristics: how your child feels about and responds to interactions with other people

All of these characteristics influence the type of learning environment that will be a good fit for your child. For example, if your child is hypersensitive to visual and auditory stimulation, then an environment where there's a lot to see (people, objects, pictures, lights, screens, etc.) and a lot to hear (voices, devices, music, traffic, etc.) may be overstimulating. But if your child tends to be less responsive to sensory stimulation, these might be welcome features of a classroom or therapy environment. If your child's movement pattern is to run, climb, jump, or dart from place to place in large open spaces, then an optimal environment for learning may be a small room where movement can be contained, but with access to a larger space for breaks. If your child processes visual information more readily than auditory information, as many autistic children do, then their environment should have appropriate forms of visual communication ready for use (such as paper, whiteboards, and other visual materials). Many autistic children are distracted or overstimulated when there's a lot of spoken language in their environment, so minimizing exposure to unnecessary spoken language (like side conversations) may be helpful. If your child responds to groups of people by withdrawing or becoming emotionally dysregulated, then one-to-one instruction may be best. But if your child gets energized and motivated by interacting with peers, then learning alongside other children in a group setting may improve their progress.

An essential aspect of strengths-based intervention for autism is to create a warm and caring atmosphere where a child feels comfortable, welcomed, and accepted. This has as much to do with the physical environment as it does with the interpersonal environment, which is the way a child is regarded and treated by others. If your child doesn't feel a basic sense of safety, security, and positivity in an environment, they may develop coping mechanisms. Some common ones include engaging in repetitive behaviors, leaving the space they're expected to stay in, making sounds, tuning out, not following instructions, and having a meltdown. A strengths-based approach and a good person-environment fit make these behaviors less likely.

Other elements that contribute to a strengths-based approach are fostering one-on-one relationships with adults and peers, using multiple learning strategies, rewarding effort, and recognizing progress. All these steps empower children to use their strengths, which builds hope and confidence and leads to greater developmental progress.

Since your child spends time in many different settings where learning can take place, the steps you and others take to appropriately modify the environment to build on strengths will make a big difference.

Here are some examples of environment modifications that I've seen help children in school, in therapy sessions, in the community, and at home:

- For twelve-year-old Ethan, finding a school environment that fit his sensory and emotional profile was key to his success in middle school. He started sixth grade at a large public middle school with nearly one thousand students. At drop-off, his parents noticed he would walk in small circles waiting for the school gates to open, surrounded by crowds of classmates. As he waited in the noisy crowd, he would engage in self-talk, repeating lines from his favorite movies. They knew this was a sign of anxiety. His classes often included thirty or more students. Ethan developed a new behavior of removing his clothes and running out of the room. They knew that Ethan had auditory sensitivity (loud noises bothered him, especially in crowds) and tactile sensitivity (he could wear only certain shirts and pants and would take off his clothes when anxious), so these new behaviors were a sign that the school environment was causing increased anxiety. They transferred Ethan to a charter school where his new classroom had twelve students and he could take frequent breaks outdoors. Ethan's anxiety and behavior soon improved.

- For eight-year-old Jessica, whose motivation and attention improved around peers, bringing other children into her therapy sessions improved her level of participation and pace of progress.

- For six-year-old Marshall, who loved to play basketball, team practices and games were overwhelming, and he had difficulty following instructions and had frequent meltdowns. His parents switched him to small-group lessons with a coach and two other boys. He was able to enjoy basketball and improve his basketball skills. The following year he rejoined the basketball league and did great in practices and games.

- Five-year-old Wendy's parents loved to have big family gatherings at their home. Wendy enjoyed these social events, too, but she became more and more hyperactive as the event went on and would often have a meltdown toward the end. Her parents tried taking Wendy to her bedroom for regular breaks every half hour and found that this helped her self-regulation and allowed her to enjoy the social gatherings without having a meltdown.

A strengths-based approach means paying attention to how your child responds in different environments and making adjustments that promote participation and learning. A strengths-based approach also involves recognizing and cultivating many types of intelligence in your child. You'll learn how to do this in the next chapter.

Chapter 4

BEYOND IQ

Recognizing Your Child's Intelligence

Intelligence is a deceptively simple word. Many people think the meaning is obvious, but coming up with a clear definition isn't easy. Over the past century neuroscientists, psychologists, and other professionals looking to understand human cognition have conducted thousands of studies and proposed a variety of definitions and assessments. Today, what *intelligence* means and how to measure it continue to be topics of debate.

This matters for you and your child because how we define *intelligence* and other abilities determines how your child's development is measured and tracked. It influences how test results are interpreted and how decisions about services are made. Because resources available for assessment differ widely from place to place, and professionals have varying degrees of training and experience, your grasp of the fundamentals will help ensure that your child's intelligence is recognized and nurtured.

Rethinking Intelligence

The word *intelligence* comes from the Latin verb *intelligere*, which means "to perceive" or "to comprehend." People often use *intelligent* to mean "smart," also a word with many meanings. Some people associate intelligence with a high level of achievement at school or work, but being intelligent doesn't rely on achieving anything. Intelligence can also refer to self-awareness and be used to distinguish humans from other species. In the digital era intelligence has been conceptualized as a computational capacity within the human brain that enables information processing.

These examples only scratch the surface. Intelligence is a concept that can refer to any mental activity related to perceiving and comprehending information, retaining information as knowledge, applying knowledge to engage in one's environment, learning from past experience, problem-solving, reasoning, and overcoming obstacles. So intelligence encompasses a wide range of dynamic capabilities.

I find it most useful to think of intelligence as the ability to acquire and use knowledge and skills. This ability can fluctuate depending on factors in the environment. As you've probably noticed, your child's performance varies depending on what they're doing, who is with them, what's happening around them, and how their performance is evaluated. People in the environment can be a particular source of stress. Autistic author and Rhodes scholar Jory Fleming says, "Anywhere there are people, it's going to be hard to find a hospitable environment for autism." And Fleming tells us that this can make it harder to communicate. "In a stressful environment, language and speech would be one of the first things to go. . . . Closing down communication language-wise actually protects my mind and my ability to think." Light, noise, smells, and other sensory stimuli can also affect an autistic person's ability to understand information and engage in their environment.

When you think of intelligence as the ability to acquire and use knowledge and skills, and recognize that this ability varies depending on factors in the environment, you can see that your child demonstrates intelligence every day, even under stressful circumstances. As you get better at recognizing this, you'll discover more opportunities to build on their intelligence. It might be by strengthening their ability to make sense of information in the environment, to engage with the world around them, or to overcome obstacles. Throughout each day, moment-to-moment, autistic people overcome obstacles and display exceptional intelligence that deserves recognition.

The Trouble with IQ

People often make the mistake of equating intelligence with IQ (intelligence quotient). In the early 1900s the French psychologist Alfred Binet invented the first "intelligence test" and with it IQ. The purpose of the test was to help the French government identify children who might need additional support to progress in their education. The test contained thirty items that ranged from copying a drawing to repeating a series of numbers to understanding a story. A child's IQ score was calculated on the basis of their performance on these test items.

Binet stated three key principles about intelligence testing.

1) Intelligence is too complex to capture with a single numerical score. A child's IQ offers a limited view intended only to direct educational assistance and does not reflect an intrinsic or permanent biological characteristic.

2) IQ serves as a rough scale and should not be used for ranking children. He intended for his scale to identify children "in order to help and improve, not to label in order to limit."

3) He insisted the emphasis should always be improvement through education. He believed that intelligence could be increased through education and that everyone could improve with support.

Unfortunately, what Binet feared might happen did happen. Over the years, practitioners and institutions far and wide have treated intelligence as a quantifiable biological attribute, like height or weight, and have used IQ and similar measures to rank and classify people. Contrary to its initial intent, intelligence testing has led to what Harvard biologist Stephen J. Gould calls the "mismeasure" of human ability.

IQ tests don't come anywhere close to capturing a person's complete mental capabilities. IQ tests and other cognitive assessments are also administered under conditions that often don't suit the sensory, language, and motor features of autistic children. So standard approaches to developmental assessment are limited when it comes to effectively assessing intelligence in autistic children. Despite this, around one-third to one-half of autistic children are given a diagnosis of intellectual disability because their cognitive abilities are estimated to be within the bottom 2.5 percent, compared with those of their same-age peers. About twenty years ago the formal medical diagnosis for these children was changed from mental retardation to intellectual disability. The negativity and stigma around the term *mental retardation* was so profound that President Barack Obama even issued an executive order banning it from all federal materials, even before the change was made in the medical field. The change was well intended—few would argue with removing such a problematic and viciously used term. But the basis of the diagnosis—whether we call it mental retardation or intellectual disability—is still flawed. And even though Binet said that a low IQ score should be used *only* as an indicator that a child will benefit from educational support, it's often used to label a child as incapable of progress and to deny essential services. That's why, in its current form, a diagnosis of intellectual disability can harm more than it helps.

Multiple Intelligences

Fortunately, other theories challenge the century-old, one-dimensional view of intelligence. One of the most influential is psychologist Howard Gardner's theory of multiple intelligences. According to Gardner, people have the capacity for different kinds of intelligence, and he identifies eight types: logical-mathematical, spatial, bodily-kinesthetic, musical, linguistic, social, intrapersonal (knowledge of oneself), and naturalist (the ability to make sense of diversity in the natural world). He proposes that human mental capacity is best considered a "collection of aptitudes" composed of these multiple intelligences and potentially others. Gardner emphasizes the importance of recognizing and nurturing "all of the varied human intelligences and all of the combinations." A shining example of musical intelligence comes from the singer and *Britain's Got Talent* winner Susan Boyle, who was mistakenly diagnosed with brain damage as a child. She later learned that her true diagnosis was autism. Daniel Tammet is an autistic adult with extraordinary mathematical and linguistic intelligence, who also had epilepsy starting in childhood. Tammet speaks seven languages and holds the European record for recalling the mathematical constant pi to the furthest decimal point—22,514 decimal places. Although he's never been able to hold a nine-to-five job, he's been able to set up his own business creating online courses in language learning and math. These are just two examples of intelligence that aren't captured by IQ.

Gardner urges us to rethink not only the meaning of *intelligence* but also how we approach assessments. He believes the results of assessments are more meaningful when children are assessed through multiple observations instead of during a single test session. He also recommends using a variety of rich materials within a child's own environment rather than the sparse, clinical environment typically used for intelligence testing. Thanks to the work of Gardner and others, more professionals are beginning to recognize the importance of changing how we assess children's abilities, including shifting from one assessment in one setting to several assessments in different settings, especially when ongoing services like developmental and behavioral therapies may be needed. Ongoing observation is now more common than it used to be, and that's a step in the right direction.

Autistic Intelligence

As far back as the 1940s we've known that certain extraordinary abilities could be part of autism. When Dr. Leo Kanner first proposed autism as a new diagnosis, he described "excellent memory" and "astounding vocabulary" as two specific examples among the children he'd seen. Films, books, and articles over the years have featured examples of autistic people with savant-type skills—also called special isolated skills—in music, math, reading, and many other areas. Kim Peek, who inspired the film *Rain Man*, could read and memorize books by scanning the left page with his left eye and the right page with his right eye. He could recall contents from over twelve thousand books with topics ranging from history to geography to sports and beyond. Leslie Lemke and Derek Paravicini, concert pianists who've been featured on the news show *60 Minutes*, can play advanced piano compositions after hearing them just once. Max Park has set multiple world records in speedcubing, a competitive sport that involves solving puzzles like the Rubik's cube. Stephen Wiltshire, the artist featured in the documentary film *Fragments of Genius*, draws complex scenes with complete accuracy from memory. Following a ten-minute helicopter ride over London, he was able to complete a detailed and perfectly scaled aerial drawing of a four-square-mile area, including over two hundred buildings. The number of autistic people with a special isolated skill varies from 10 percent to as high as 71 percent, depending on the types and levels of skill that are included.

Recently, researchers have expanded their exploration beyond the category of special skills to look at other unique cognitive abilities in autism. In *The Pattern Seekers: How Autism Drives Human Invention*, psychologist Simon Baron-Cohen explains that the autistic brain is hypertuned to analyze patterns and systems. A child carrying out repetitive behavior, like flipping on and off a light switch or opening and closing a door, may not seem to have a clear purpose. But the child is actually examining the environment, motivated by curiosity for how things work. Details in the environment that many overlook, like how doors open or how lights turn on, can capture the interest of an autistic child. Repetitive behaviors can be a child's way of experimenting in their environment to explore if-then relationships or how actions lead to responses. The drive to understand causal relationships like these can lead to new systems and inventions.

The autistic mind is a curious mind experimenting with the environment, and experimentation requires repetition to fully examine whether patterns hold under different conditions and whether they continue to remain true over time. Baron-Cohen says, "A child's relentless experimenting and detailed observations are the product of a mind whose pattern-seeking engine operates in overdrive and can lead them to invent, and sometimes to become great inventors." He says that though we don't know for certain whether Albert Einstein would have been diagnosed with autism based on how we understand it today, we know that he showed many autistic features, including a pattern-seeking mind that made him a great scientist and inventor.

Is your own brain attracted to analyzing patterns and systems? See if you respond yes to these statements from Simon Baron-Cohen's questionnaire called Systemizing Quotient–Revised:

- When I learn about a new category, I like to go into detail to understand the small differences between different members of that category.

- I am interested in knowing the path a river takes from its course to the sea.

- When traveling by train, I often wonder exactly how the rail networks are coordinated.

- I enjoy looking through product catalogs to see the details of each product and how it compares with others.

- When I look at a mountain, I think about how precisely it was formed.

- When I learn a language, I become intrigued by its grammatical rules.

- When I listen to a piece of music, I always notice the way it's structured.

We know that repetitive behaviors and restricted interests can reflect a pattern-seeking mind. They can also represent other ways of making sense of the world. In the book *Autistic Intelligence*, sociologists Douglas W. Maynard and Jason Turowetz explain that autistic people reason, make decisions, and act in purposeful ways based on their experience in the world. The autistic author Tito Mukhopadhyay, for example, writes that the reason he spins while looking at a rotating fan is because he sees the spinning blades become unified into one thing. He experiences his own body as scattered and difficult to unify, so spinning helps him bring his body together and feel whole.

Other autistic authors also offer rationale for behaviors that may at first seem unusual. In his book *Look Me in the Eye*, John Elder Robison explains why he says "Woof!" when he needs to start a conversation or fill a silence. He's learned from experience that when he starts a conversation or responds to someone else, what he says can be perceived as rude or surprising, especially if he says something true that others don't necessarily want to hear. He tells us, "That's why I learned some years ago to utter a noncommittal 'Woof!' if I need to begin a conversation or fill a silence. People hear that and are not sure what to say, but they don't usually perceive a woof as rude." Another example comes from Naoki Higashida, author of *The Reason I Jump*. He explains that he cups his ears because there are certain noises that other people may not notice that can cause him discomfort and fear. He says, "It feels as if the ground is shaking and the landscape around us starts coming to get us, and it's absolutely terrifying. So cupping our ears is a measure we take to protect ourselves and get back our grip on where we are." These examples show us how behaviors that might be labeled as maladaptive are, in fact, intelligent ways of navigating the environment.

Some autistic people have described what it's like when they engage their intellect. Higashida says:

I do understand things, but my way of remembering them works differently from everyone else's. I imagine a normal person's memory is arranged continuously, like a line. My memory, however, is more like a pool of dots. I'm always 'picking up' these dots—by asking my questions—so I can arrive back at the memory that the dots represent.

Jory Fleming describes his intellect in this way:

I work with data points. They contain information and look like little beads. I put things in these beads. It could be anything from something I've read in a book to something a professor or a friend has said. Or it could be an observation that I've made—something that was never based in words in the first place. But even if there was language in there at some point, I've removed the language by placing it inside the bead. All the beads are the same, and I treat them all the same. I take whatever knowledge is being processed and put it into Jory format.

He can move these beads around in his mind to change their position in his "mind space" and he can draw connections between beads. To retrieve information he searches through the beads: "I have to scan the whole thing—it's not even organized by areas; rather, when I start thinking about something, my brain does a complete scan. A very tiny fraction of my brain is actively looking at each bead and deciding yes, no, yes, no." Using his unique style of thinking, he explains, he was able to improve his social-emotional intelligence. As part of a college seminar on how to serve as a peer leader, he received a manual on how to respond to other people who are in emotional distress. He memorized this step-by-step guide and was able to retrieve and implement the instructions just as they'd been explicitly defined in the manual. By doing so, he mastered a task that any person would find daunting—to support others in states of emotional crisis.

Fleming's description of how he experiences and manages emotions reflects what could be considered a unique form of autistic emotional intelligence. He experiences a range of emotions, but he's able to observe them at a distance so that he isn't overcome or distressed by them. He says, "Emotions seem to be happening further away from me." For this reason, emotions don't govern his responses to others, and he doesn't hold on to negative feelings. With respect to heated reactions that people have toward other people who disagree with them, especially on social media, he says, "Having a reaction just because another person says something that I disagree with wouldn't occur." In this way Fleming displays skills reminiscent of those that advanced meditators and spiritual leaders spend years cultivating. He contrasts his experience of emotions with the way emotions can take hold of neurotypical people, fueling negativity and obstructing productive dialogue. Fleming is the first to acknowledge that there's no single autistic experience, just as there's no single neurotypical experience. But the insights he offers are invaluable in helping to expand how we think about the wide variety of autistic abilities.

Verbal ability may represent yet another type of autistic intelligence. Researchers have found that language skills, both spoken and written, develop in a different sequence in autistic children than in neurotypical children. Since speaking is not necessary for verbal skills like reading, writing, and sign language, a child who does not speak may be called nonspeaking but should not be called nonverbal, since the child may understand language and may have skills for reading, writing, or sign language. Neurotypical children babble, then develop one- and two-word phrases, then speak in sentences, and then learn to read. In autistic children these steps often occur in a different order and some are skipped entirely. Autistic children often recognize letters and numbers before they develop basic speech. Comprehension of complex written material can also come before the development of fluent speech. Hyperlexia, the precocious ability to read before age five without formal teaching, is increasingly recognized as an early sign of autism and happens more frequently in children with delayed speech. So we now know that many autistic children learn to read before they learn to speak, and even those who speak may prefer written over oral communication. Unfortunately, many speech-language services haven't adapted to this new understanding of autistic language development and are still using approaches based on neurotypical development. But use of written language earlier in a child's therapy program is beginning to make its way into early intervention services for autism. If you see signs of hyperlexia in your own child, you can work with your therapy team to include reading and writing early in your child's program.

The "Just-Right Challenge"

Knowing that autistic minds work differently, that they have unique forms of intelligence and distinctive developmental paths, how do you give your child the best support for learning?

The answer comes from the work of Dr. A. Jean Ayres, an occupational therapist and educational psychologist. Ayres's pioneering work in child development has revolutionized our understanding of how to help children learn. Over several decades she developed an approach to therapy based on understanding a child's sensory perceptions. Prior to her work very little had been done to explore how differences in processing sensory information could affect a child's learning and behavior. We now understand that all learning relies on the ability to perceive and process information coming from our senses. Ayres helped us understand that how the brain translates sensory information into motor action is crucial for all learning and behavior. So when we support the development of sensory and motor systems, learning and behavior can improve.

In her work Ayres emphasized the importance of identifying the "just-right challenge." She described this as a task slightly above a child's current skill level. With support, the child can carry out the task, and with additional practice, the child can complete it independently. The just-right challenge creates an optimal situation for learning and allows a child to go just beyond their current performance level without experiencing frustration. Ayres wrote, "When the optimum-for-growth situation is achieved, the child 'turns on' [showing a] zest for experience." The person working with the child, whether a therapist, teacher, parent, or other partner, creates the just-right challenge by arranging the environment and providing guidance. This type of informed guidance is sometimes called "scaffolding," because it's a structure that supports a child's learning, just as physical scaffolding supports the construction of a new building.

Creating these optimal learning moments for your child means understanding your child's current skills in each of the major developmental domains:

- Sensory
- Motor
- Cognitive
- Language
- Social
- Emotional

Therapists and other professionals can partner with you to arrive at an understanding of your child's current development and show you how to create the just-right challenge for your child in everyday activities. In part 2, I'll also provide you with exercises to get you on the right track.

In group settings like classrooms, creating the just-right challenge for every child is a tough job. Because school systems need to provide education to many students, class sizes are often large, and instructors rely on standardized curricula that usually aren't tailored to the strengths of autistic children, even in special education classrooms. This means that your child may not receive many opportunities in school to experience the just-right challenge. Your knowledge in this area, and the support of skilled therapists who can provide individual or small-group instruction, will ensure that your child gets to experience the just-right challenge frequently and all the rich learning those moments bring.

Once we recognize the many forms intelligence can take, we see that terms like *high-functioning* and *low-functioning*, commonly used in autism, aren't helpful. These labels imply that we can group autistic people into two categories of function, when we know there are far more dimensions to someone's abilities. A better option is to think about how much support could benefit your child. This means looking at your child's neurodevelopmental profile; considering the support being provided at school, at home, in a clinic setting, and in the community; and determining whether additional support could be helpful. It's important to keep in mind that this is dynamic and that all people, whether neurotypical or neurodivergent, benefit from varying levels of support as they grow and as circumstances change. The ultimate goal is to help your child move from higher to lower levels of support over time as their abilities grow.

Now that you're thinking in terms of your child's strengths and intelligence and have a holistic view of their development, you can move forward with building the components of a whole-child program. Part 2 of this book guides you through the five key elements of the whole-child path: brain-body health, development, behavior, family, and community.

Part 2

THE WHOLE-CHILD PATH

The path you'll learn about here is one I've traveled with thousands of families. From the moment of diagnosis through the days, months, and years ahead, the path brings connection, learning, fulfillment, and joy. But there's also the possibility of detours along the way that can lead to fear, stress, isolation, and loss of hope. Each time a new family walks into my office, I see the potential for these experiences on the road ahead.

What makes the difference is a combination of mindset, knowledge, and support. You're already well on your way there. In part 1, you learned the key principles of fostering a holistic mindset. You learned that your child is neurodivergent, multidimensional, strong, and intelligent. You learned how to see your whole child and how to understand all of autism.

In part 2, I explain how to navigate the five key elements of the whole-child path:

1. Brain-Body Health

Everything your child does, including how your child engages with others and the world around them, reflects the brain in action. Your child's health across all body systems supports the brain to function at its best. You'll learn about the latest tests and therapies for genetic, metabolic, neurological, gastrointestinal, and other conditions that co-occur with autism.

2. Development

Your child develops new abilities by forming brain networks for sensory, motor, cognitive, language, social, and emotional abilities. You'll learn how to support brain development "from the inside" through nutrition, exercise, and stress reduction. You'll also learn how to support brain development "from the outside" by making the most of professional therapy services and by creating the just-right challenge for your child in everyday routines, which is the most effective way to build brain networks.

3. Behavior

Behavior is a broad term that refers to just about anything a person says or does. But in autism the meaning of *behavior* is closely connected to the science of behaviorism, which looks at how a person's behavior changes when the people, objects, and events around them change. You'll learn how to positively influence your child's behavior by changing their surroundings and experiences.

4. Family

The well-being of each family member matters for your child's health, but all too often it's neglected. You'll learn steps to improve health and wellness in family members and to improve peace, stability, and happiness at home.

5. Community

All children need places outside the home where they can feel comfortable and be themselves. Finding those places can transform your child's outlook on life and willingness to take on new challenges. Positive experiences in the community are where autistic people most often describe finding inspiration and purpose.

What all autistic children have in common is the need for attention to these five elements. Where all children differ is how each element should be navigated—which assessments and therapies should be done, in what order, and what steps to take based on assessment results and your child's response to therapies. Successfully navigating the path means honoring your child's unique differences as well as their similarities to other autistic children.

This path is stepwise. Any action, like completing a blood test or starting a new therapy, can lead to findings that determine what the next steps should be. Even though you can't map the trip from start to finish, you can make the best decisions at each point on the journey by paying attention to what your child is showing you.

The path is generous with opportunities for learning, discovery, and joy. But there are potential hazards, too. As you probably know, an internet search brings up thousands of so-called treatments for autism, and the pull to enter the rabbit hole can be strong. Putting resources in the wrong places or focusing on only one element while neglecting others can make the journey harder. But remember that even in the most difficult moments, there's a positive way forward.

No matter what's happened until now—what's worked or what hasn't, the progress or the plateaus, the struggles or the successes— you can start fresh with all the tools for navigating the whole-child path with confidence.

Chapter 5

AUTISM PLUS (+)

Improving Brain and Body Health

Jacob was a sweet, quiet baby who rarely made a fuss. But around his first birthday, his mom noticed he didn't look at her when she called his name, and by eighteen months, he still didn't say any words. His pediatrician referred him to a speech-language therapist and he made good progress. By age two he could say phrases like "big ball" and "more cars." His language continued to grow, but his mom noticed he didn't interact with children at the playground and instead lined up toys or ran his fingers through the sand. He became picky about the food he would eat and was often constipated.

After Jacob's third birthday, they moved to a new city to be closer to family, and his mom gave birth to Jacob's baby brother. Though he'd always been a good sleeper, Jacob started waking several times a night, which his parents thought was because of the changes at home. At his four-year checkup, his pediatrician recommended a developmental evaluation with a psychologist at the local children's hospital. The family waited six months for the next available appointment. At that appointment a psychologist diagnosed Jacob with autism and referred him for behavior therapy and occupational therapy.

Both therapies had a six-month waitlist. By then Jacob was four and a half years old.

To his parents' alarm, after one year of therapies, Jacob's development hadn't improved, and in some areas he'd regressed. His behavior therapist suggested that he see a doctor to explore medications. His parents thought it over, talked to other parents, and researched options online. They decided it was too soon to start medications—Jacob was still so young. So they didn't schedule a medical consultation.

Then one morning his parents found him in bed with his body shaking and called 911. An electroencephalogram (EEG) done at the hospital confirmed seizure activity, and they started him on medication. The family met with me the following week for follow-up care, and I immediately conducted the blood, urine, and saliva tests for co-occurring genetic and metabolic conditions. At that point Jacob was five and a half years old.

Even though Jacob first showed signs of autism when he was one year old, he didn't receive the appropriate medical testing until he was five and a half. His test results showed that he had a genetic condition leading to a malfunction in a key metabolic pathway. With medication therapy for his seizures and nutritional changes to address his metabolic condition, Jacob began to make progress in all his therapies.

Unfortunately, delays like this in medical care for autism are the rule, not the exception. An autism diagnosis usually comes years after the first signs of autism appear. The wait for an autism diagnostic evaluation alone can be up to eighteen months. After the diagnosis is made, the focus usually shifts to starting therapy services. Most children don't receive the appropriate evaluation for co-occurring medical conditions until many years later, and some don't receive it at all.

As you've probably experienced firsthand, autism care is fragmented, which means children get pieces of care from different providers. Every transition from one provider to another brings delays in care and incomplete communication. In Jacob's case, the professionals he saw early on weren't equipped to explain why medical care was important. Even in cases where parents know to seek medical care, the wait time to see medical specialists who can perform appropriate tests is usually three to twelve months unless a child has an acute event like a seizure. These are among the longest wait times in all of medicine. Yet another barrier is the cost of medical tests. Insurers may not cover the cost of certain tests or may have strict requirements that delay access.

Other brain conditions have faced similar challenges in getting people to recognize the need for rapid access to medical care. The phrase "time is brain" was created to help drive home the message that when it comes to neurological conditions, time lost can mean brain lost. The most notable example comes from stroke, which involves the acute loss of blood flow to part of the brain. Health outcomes for stroke have improved by educating and improving awareness among providers and the public. Clear management protocols and rigorous measurement of the time from symptom onset to appropriate diagnosis and treatment have led to vast improvements in care. Even though what's happening in the brain in autism is not the same as what's happening in stroke, a similar approach can help change the status quo so that children get appropriate medical care as soon as autism is diagnosed.

An Autism Diagnosis Is a Starting Point

Autism describes a set of social and behavioral characteristics but it's not a specific biological diagnosis. It tells us about a person's behavior but not about what's happening in their body. In fact, we know that many different biological subgroups fall under the diagnostic umbrella of autism. Researchers have tried to define a clear set of biological subgroups or "subtypes" of autism, but it's been challenging because there are so many biological differences within the autism diagnostic umbrella. Some people have no genetic, metabolic, neurological, gastrointestinal, or other co-occurring conditions, while others have many. From what we can tell from research so far, there isn't a simple way to group autism into specific biological subtypes. So the best approach we have right now is to consider each child as their own unique biological subtype. That's why it's so important to understand that an autism diagnosis is the beginning, not the end, of the diagnostic process. From there, the goal is to learn more about your child's biology and use that information to individualize their care.

An autism diagnosis is based on what others observe about your child's behavior. It can be compared with observing someone who's limping. The limp could be from a broken bone, torn ligament, sore muscle, pinched nerve, or brain tumor. No one would think to diagnose a limp and stop there without providing a thorough physical examination and appropriate testing. It's time we recognize the same is needed for autism.

Treatable Causes of Developmental Symptoms

It's important to pause here to recognize that when we use the word *treatment* in relation to autism, we're referring to the treatment of co-occurring medical conditions and not to autism itself. Many autistic people feel that autism is an important part of their identity, in a similar way that one experiences gender, religious, or cultural identity. We should not label that identity as needing medical treatment. In fact, the idea that aspects of a person's identity have a biological cause that should be fixed or cured can be extremely harmful. The medical field has frequently made this mistake in the past, so we need to be careful not to repeat it.

It's important to honor autistic identity *and* provide high quality health-care services. The two are not at odds. This means that autistic intelligence and other strengths should be recognized and nurtured. At the same time, if co-occurring medical conditions are affecting a child's health, we need to diagnose them as quickly as possible and offer appropriate treatments.

The group of co-occurring medical conditions that deserves the most urgent attention is the one that doctors and researchers refer to as *treatable causes*. For about 5 percent of autistic children, medical testing reveals a specific treatable metabolic or neurological condition that's directly causing developmental delay or regression. The two main categories of treatable causes are *metabolic disorders* and *epileptic encephalopathies* (pronounced en-sefə-LOP-ə-theez).

METABOLIC DISORDERS

When we hear the word *metabolism*, we often think of weight loss, but its meaning is much broader than that. *Metabolism* refers to the thousands and thousands of chemical processes that take place in the body to maintain life. Another way to think of metabolism is how the body converts nutrients into energy for all its functions and gets rid of unnecessary, potentially toxic waste products that are created in the process.

Many medical conditions affect metabolism, but the group of metabolic disorders that we're talking about here are those caused by a single gene mutation that a person is born with. Research studies have identified at least thirty metabolic disorders of this kind that can lead to autism. A child is more likely to have one of these metabolic disorders if they have a diagnosis of epilepsy; a higher degree of developmental delay in sensory, motor, cognitive, social, or language domains; distinctive facial or other physical features; or medical diagnoses in other body systems, such as gastrointestinal, hormonal, or other systems.

In the United States and many other countries, the blood screen done on newborns at the time of birth tests for many metabolic disorders. Depending on your child's medical history and physical exam, a neurologist or geneticist can determine whether additional tests, like blood, urine, or saliva tests, are needed. Effective treatments for these conditions range from making changes to the diet, supplementing with vitamins or other nutrients, or treatment with enzymes or other medications. When a child has a metabolic disorder, early diagnosis and effective treatment can make a tremendous difference in their health and development.

EPILEPTIC ENCEPHALOPATHIES

Epilepsy is a neurological condition characterized by recurrent seizures. Seizures are episodes in which neurons in the brain fire in an atypical way. Usually seizures lead to involuntary movements and to changes in a person's level of consciousness. But some seizures are more subtle and may cause only a brief interruption to a person's usual behavior or may be completely undetectable (sometimes called "silent seizures").

In children, epilepsy can sometimes disrupt the course of brain development, causing delay or regression in language, cognitive, motor, or social skills, and this can happen with or without observable seizures. These forms of epilepsy, called epileptic encephalopathies, are uncommon and represent only a small minority of epilepsy diagnoses in autistic and neurotypical children, but they are important to know about. A child may receive an autism diagnosis and the underlying epileptic encephalopathy may remain undiagnosed unless an electroencephalogram is done to measure the brain's electrical activity. Effective treatment of epileptic encephalopathy can in some instances lead to dramatic developmental gains, so it's important to work with a neurologist to determine if seizures are occurring and, if so, to explore treatment options.

Diagnosing and Treating Other Co-occurring Medical Conditions

Many medical conditions co-occur with autism, and knowing about these conditions is important to ensure that your child receives appropriate care. Each of these areas represents an opportunity to deepen your understanding of your child's unique biology and to take action to improve your child's health and development.

You'll see there are many different treatments available for autism's co-occurring conditions, which means there are many ways to help your child, but it can also feel overwhelming. It may help to know they all fall into one of the following categories, and you can use these categories to organize your approach:

- *Lifestyle changes,* like making changes to daily routines or increasing physical exercise
- *Dietary changes,* like adding and/or removing certain foods from your child's diet

- **Nutritional supplements,** like giving your child certain vitamins, minerals, or other dietary supplements
- **Medications,** including both over-the-counter and prescription medications
- **Neuromodulation therapies (or device therapies),** like technology that delivers electrical or magnetic stimulation to the brain or that uses software to engage a child in therapeutic activities on a computer or tablet
- **Developmental and behavioral approaches,** like speech-language therapy, occupational therapy, physical therapy, music therapy, behavior therapy, counseling, or others

One reason these categories are helpful is that they show you the range of options you can choose from to support your child. Some families prefer to start with lifestyle changes and developmental or behavioral approaches. Others may have been doing those for years and are ready to explore medications. Sometimes medication is needed early on so that a child can participate in and benefit from developmental or behavioral therapies. Some families find dietary changes easy to implement but others find them stressful. Some families want to do it all at once, while others prefer to start with one category and gradually layer in others. The best approach for your child is one that you feel comfortable and capable carrying through.

GENETIC CONDITIONS

In just the past decade researchers have published over ten thousand studies on the genetics of autism. Trying to understand these complex studies can make your head spin. Fortunately, what you need to know to help your child can be boiled down to a few simple facts.

When we talk about understanding your child's genetic information, we're talking about DNA. DNA is a long, ladder-shaped molecule that's located in our cells. Each rung of the ladder is made of interlocking units called bases that can come in one of four versions, each designated by a letter—A, T, G, or C—which make up what's sometimes called the DNA alphabet. These letters of the DNA alphabet are organized into sequences called genes, and genes are organized into longer pieces called chromosomes. You can think of chromosomes as cookbooks and genes as the recipes.

When I recommend genetic testing to parents, the most common question I get is "Genes can't be changed, so how can this help?" One way genetic testing can help is by revealing mutations in genes that cause metabolic disorders. Often there are effective treatments to correct the metabolic disturbance caused by the gene. So even though the gene doesn't change, its effects on the brain and body can be changed.

Another way genetic testing can help is by identifying a genetic variant that causes a specific genetic condition. Well-researched genetic conditions that co-occur with autism include Fragile X syndrome, Down syndrome, Rett syndrome, Angelman syndrome, Prader-Willi syndrome, Phelan-McDermid syndrome, tuberous sclerosis complex, and others. Not all people with these genetic conditions have autism, but many do. These genetic conditions have well developed best-practice guidelines, and researchers are actively investigating many promising treatments. Knowing if your child has one of these diagnoses allows you to connect to excellent clinical and research centers and to family support groups. After one mother received a diagnosis of Phelan-McDermid syndrome for her teenage daughter, she told me, "Now we have a tribe. And that's something we're grateful for."

Even if genetic testing doesn't reveal a metabolic disorder or another genetic condition, it still has the potential to tell us something important about your child's biology. Often genetic testing identifies variants in a person's genes and we aren't sure what they mean—the term used in medicine for this kind of genetic finding is *variants of uncertain significance.* Recently a colleague asked me to review a patient's genetic findings that showed several variants of uncertain significance. Some of these variants were in genes involved in mitochondrial function. Another variant was in a gene that regulates the flow of sodium into and out of neurons. These all serve as clues that can guide the selection of nutritional supplements, medications, and other medical therapies to support your child's behavior, development, and overall health.

So there are many ways that knowing your child's genetic information might be beneficial. We now also recognize that the environment can influence how our genes get expressed—this is called *epigenetics.* The way we live our lives—including our diet, exercise routine, stress level, and exposure to certain pollutants in the environment—has the potential to "turn on" or "turn off" genes. In chapter 6 you'll learn more about steps to improve potential epigenetic factors like nutrition, exercise, and stress.

You should also know that the technological capability to change genes does, in fact, exist today. One example that's received a lot of attention is the gene-editing technology called CRISPR. Genetic conditions have been successfully cured using CRISPR, but on a very limited basis. A number of hurdles still need to be overcome, but in the future this technology is likely to become more widely available.

There are several ways we can examine a person's genetic information:

- The genetic test called *chromosomal microarray analysis* looks at a person's chromosomes for any missing pieces (deletions) or extra pieces (duplications). This test identifies a genetic factor in about 20 percent of autistic children.

- Another genetic test called *whole exome sequencing* looks at about twenty thousand genes to find alterations to the sequence of DNA. Whole exome sequencing identifies a genetic factor in about 15 percent of autistic children.

- A genetic test that includes a subset of genes from whole exome sequencing is called a *gene panel*. The panel includes genes that are related to a set of symptoms of conditions rather than looking at all genes.

- A genetic test called *mitochondrial DNA sequencing* looks at a set of genes within tiny structures inside of cells called mitochondria. You'll learn more about mitochondria later in this chapter.

- The genetic test called *whole genome sequencing* looks at even more genes beyond those included in whole exome sequencing. Whole genome sequencing is a newer test and not yet available on a routine basis.

These tests need to be ordered by a medical professional and are done specifically to look for genetic findings associated with a medical diagnosis such as autism. Some genetic tests like 23andMe are available to do on your own, but tests like these are generally meant for people interested in learning more about their ancestry, not for people trying to understand a medical diagnosis. They look for genetic variations that are common in the general population, not ones that are specific to autism.

Experts agree that autistic children should have a chromosomal microarray analysis and testing for Fragile X syndrome. If these tests don't identify a genetic finding, and sometimes even if they do, your doctor may recommend additional tests, such as gene panels or whole exome sequencing. Some insurance plans cover these tests and others don't, so cost can sometimes be a barrier. But if your doctor feels strongly that one or more of these tests are needed, there may be low-cost or no-cost options you can pursue with a genetic testing company or by participating in a research study.

EPILEPSY

Around one in eight autistic children have epilepsy, a condition characterized by recurrent seizures. Epilepsy is about ten times more common in autistic children than in non-autistic children. Earlier in this chapter you learned about a rare category of epilepsy called epileptic encephalopathy that can cause developmental delay or regression, including features of autism. Many other types of epilepsy can also co-occur with autism, and effective treatment of these types of epilepsy can often lead to improvement in behavior, mental health, and quality of life.

The single most important thing to know about seizures is that it's not always easy to tell if a person is having one. When most people think of seizures, they think of *grand mal seizures*—what neurologists call generalized tonic-clonic seizures—which cause loss of consciousness and shaking of the whole body. But most of the time seizures are more subtle, and it's hard to know just by looking at your child if seizures are happening in the brain.

How a seizure looks and feels depends on the parts of the brain that are involved. Seizures may look like repeated movements of an arm, a leg, or another part of the body. They may look like a lapse of attention or "staring spell." In some cases there's no outward sign at all, but the person having the seizure might experience certain smells, tastes, or other sensations, or they may be completely unaware that anything unusual is happening. Seizures can occur when a person is asleep or when they're awake. The reason why seizures can look and feel so many ways is because they can happen in any localized part of the brain—these types of seizures are called *focal* or *partial* seizures. Or they can happen throughout the brain—these types of seizures are called *generalized* seizures.

Seizures can begin at any age, and they're more likely if a person also has a co-occurring genetic condition or if a part of the brain has formed differently during fetal development (called a *brain malformation*, which is diagnosed by a brain scan).

Since epilepsy is common in autism and since we can't tell if someone has seizures just by looking at them, it's important for autistic children to have an electroencephalogram (EEG). During an EEG, multiple electrodes are placed on the head to measure the brain's electrical activity. This can be done in a doctor's office, in a hospital, or at home. The goal of the EEG is to record as much information as possible while also making the experience as comfortable as possible for your child. Even though the test itself is not painful, many children find it unpleasant to lie still and have something attached to their head. An EEG is a test that might need to be repeated at regular intervals, so it's important for it to be a positive experience. In my office we provide videos and stories to let a child know what to expect. Children should have their favorite blanket, stuffed animal, pillow, book, device, snack, game, or anything else that provides comfort. Sometimes a short EEG recording of thirty minutes or less is enough to get the information needed, but other times a child might need to have an EEG recording that continues for one or more days. Your doctor will decide what's needed based on your child's medical history.

In addition to detecting seizures, an EEG recording can pick up more subtle electrical discharges that aren't seizures on their own but that indicate a part of the brain is firing in an atypical way and is prone to generating seizures. An EEG done during sleep can provide information about sleep quality and how the brain is moving through different stages of sleep. It's ideal to capture sleep during an EEG, and this can be done by taking steps to help your child fall asleep during a daytime EEG or by having an EEG done during your child's overnight sleep. About 60 percent of autistic people have atypical findings on their EEG. These findings provide valuable information to guide your child's care.

If an epilepsy diagnosis is made, you and your doctor will work together to evaluate a range of treatment options. Treatment decisions should be made by carefully considering all potential benefits and risks. Seizures are most often treated with medications, but nonmedication therapies, such as dietary interventions, an implantable device, and brain surgery, are also options for some types of epilepsy. For autistic individuals who don't have epilepsy but have atypical electrical discharges on EEG, some research studies have found that treatment using seizure medications has the potential to lead to improvements in cognitive function, behavior, and mental health. This is yet another way that EEG findings can help you to make decisions about your child's medical care.

How to Reduce Seizures

LIFESTYLE CHANGES

Sleep deprivation makes seizures more likely, so improving sleep can reduce seizures. Exercise and stress reduction can improve sleep and may also improve health in other ways that reduce seizures.

DIETARY CHANGES

For over a century, dietary changes have been used to treat epilepsy. These four diets are currently used for epilepsy treatment and should be used under the guidance of a medical provider who specializes in dietary treatment of epilepsy:

Ketogenic diet: a high-fat diet with most of a person's calories coming from fats

Modified Atkins diet: a high-fat diet that is less restrictive than the ketogenic diet

Medium-chain triglyceride diet: a diet that includes a type of fat supplement called medium-chain triglyceride oil

Low-glycemic index diet: a diet that is less restrictive than the ketogenic diet, limits daily intake of carbohydrates, and focuses on including carbohydrates that don't cause spikes in blood sugar after eating

NUTRITIONAL SUPPLEMENTS

Cannabidiol (CBD): a compound found in cannabis (marijuana) that's available as a dietary supplement or as a prescription medication and is used to treat seizures.

Vitamin B6, vitamin B7, vitamin B9, and magnesium: nutritional supplements that are sometimes used to treat specific seizure types.

MEDICATIONS

Anti-epileptic medications commonly used in autism (the generic name is followed by the brand name in parentheses):

- Lamotrigine (Lamictal): a good choice for many seizure types. For some people, it has the benefit of stabilizing mood and improving behavior.

- Oxcarbazepine (Trileptal): a good choice for focal seizure types. For some people, it has the benefit of stabilizing mood and improving behavior.
- Levetiracetam (Keppra): a good choice for many seizure types. For some people, it has the downside of increasing irritability and worsening behavior. This side effect may resolve by taking vitamin B6.

Other anti-epileptic medications that may be used in autism: brivaracetam (Briviact), carbamazepine (Tegretol), cenobamate (Xcopri), clobazam (Onfi), eslicarbazepine (Aptiom), felbamate (Felbatol), gabapentin (Neurontin), lacosamide (Vimpat), perampanel (Fycompa), phenobarbital, phenytoin (Dilantin), pregabalin (Lyrica), rufinamide (Banzel), topiramate (Topamax), valproic acid (Depakote), vigabatrin (Sabril), and zonisamide (Zonegran)

Cannabidiol is available as a prescription medication (Epidiolex).

Steroids can be used to treat certain seizure types.

Medications used to stop a seizure that's already started (sometimes called "rescue" medications): diazepam (Diastat or Valtoco), clonazepam (Klonopin), and midazolam (Nayzilam)

VAGUS NERVE STIMULATION

A device called a vagus nerve stimulator is implanted under the skin near the left side of the chest and stimulates the vagus nerve to reduce focal seizures that aren't fully controlled by medications.

EPILEPSY SURGERY

Surgery can be considered for some seizure types and requires an evaluation with an epilepsy team that has expertise in this area.

SLEEP DISTURBANCE

Sleep is as essential to life as food and water. Even though we think of sleep as a time of rest, the body is busy repairing and restoring itself. The brain is especially busy, processing what's happened during the day and storing important information as memories. Recently, researchers have discovered that during sleep the brain also cleans out waste that has built up from the day. This biological housekeeping makes the difference between waking up with brain fog or a clear mind. Over time, how well we sleep has lasting effects on our ability to think, learn, communicate, and remember.

Most of what we know about the brain during sleep comes from research over the last several decades, but the idea that sleep is a period of biological activity and not simply a state of rest has been around much longer. As the ancient Greek philosopher Heraclitus said, "Even a soul submerged in sleep is hard at work."

Between 50 and 80 percent of autistic children have trouble getting to sleep or staying asleep. Sometimes the reason is a co-occurring medical condition, like epilepsy, heartburn (also called acid reflux), or an obstruction to the upper airway (which can lead to snoring and a condition called sleep apnea). Discomfort anywhere in the body, including a toothache, headache, earache, stomachache, skin irritation, sore throat, or allergy symptoms can all disrupt sleep. These are more likely to go undetected if a child isn't able to describe what they're feeling. For some children, trouble sleeping is caused by aspects of the environment, like lighting, noise, or temperature. For others, it can be caused by habits that develop over time, like going to find a parent in the middle of the night or resisting falling asleep alone. Researchers have found biological differences in autistic children that can also contribute to sleep difficulties, like differences in brain chemicals and hormones, including serotonin (a neurotransmitter that influences mood and sleep), melatonin (a hormone that helps control the sleep-wake cycle), and cortisol (a hormone involved in the body's response to stress).

Whatever the cause or causes may be, there are many ways to help. For most children this means making a number of changes to daytime activities, the bedtime routine, and the sleep environment. Your doctor may also recommend certain medical tests, like an EEG, sleep study, or blood tests. Sometimes changes to the diet, adding nutritional supplements, or starting a medication can help. The one thing that enables all of these steps to go well is your positive energy and mental clarity. That's why it's essential to make sure *you're* getting enough sleep. As you learn about creating a sleep improvement plan for your child, you can apply any of the steps to enhance your own sleep, too.

Sleep Improvement Plan

How much sleep a person needs is highly individual. There's no magic number that works for everyone. Most preschool-age children need about eleven to thirteen hours of sleep a day, including naps. School-age children need about nine to eleven hours, and teens need about eight to nine hours of sleep each day. Signs of sleepiness during the day, like yawning, drowsiness, and irritability, probably mean that your child would benefit from better sleep. Working with a doctor is important to determine whether medical conditions might be interfering with your child's sleep, but there are many steps you can take on your own, too.

First, get a full picture of your child's sleep by tracking daytime activities, the bedtime routine, and other information for several days using a worksheet like this one:

Date: _____

DURING THE DAY

Exercise: _____

_____

Naps: _____

_____

Outdoor activities: _____

_____

Caffeine intake: _____

_____

Sugary foods: _____

_____

DURING THE EVENING

Bedtime routine: start time _____ p.m.

Describe the sequence of activities leading up to bedtime: _____

_____

_____

Describe the sleep setting: _____

_____

_____

NIGHTTIME

What time your child got in bed with lights off: _____ p.m.

What time your child fell asleep: _____ p.m.

Describe any strategies you used to help your child fall asleep:

_____

_____

_____

_____

Describe any night wakings (how many, what time they occurred, how long they lasted, what your child did when they woke up, and how you responded): _____

_____

_____

_____

_____

MORNING

What time your child woke up in the morning to start the day: _____ a.m.

Once you've taken a record of your child's sleep, look for opportunities to make improvements in any of these areas:

Daytime Activities

- Add physical exercise and other activities that move the body and increase the heart rate. More physical activity during the day promotes better sleep at night.

- Increase the time your child spends outdoors in natural sunlight, especially during the morning and early afternoon. This helps regulate hormones in the body that promote a healthy sleep-wake cycle.

- Reduce stress and exposure to events that may increase anxiety. These kinds of experiences activate the body's stress response and can make sleep more difficult.

- Keep an eye on the amount of time your child naps during the day. Shorten naptime or discontinue napping if your child doesn't seem to need it. Try to end naps by 4 p.m.

- Eliminate food and drinks that contain caffeine.

Evening and Bedtime Activities

- Before bedtime, reduce activities that are physically or mentally stimulating, like playing sports, doing homework, playing video games, and other exciting or energizing activities. The evening should be a time to settle down and begin preparing for sleep.

- Add relaxing activities, like listening to calming music, reading, listening to stories, taking a warm bath, or engaging in quiet play activities. What helps one child relax may not help another, so adapt the evening routine to include those things that are relaxing for you and your child. If bath time is energizing, move it to another time of day.

- If your child gets hungry at bedtime or during the night, consider a small evening snack. Try to choose a snack that has more protein, fat, and complex carbohydrates, rather than one that mainly provides simple carbohydrates. Some good choices include foods with whole grains, avocado, nuts or nut butter, hummus, beans, or eggs.

- Reduce bright lights and screen time. These can suppress levels of melatonin in the brain and make it harder to sleep.

- Keep a consistent bedtime routine that includes simple activities that lead up to sleep, like changing into pajamas, brushing teeth, using the toilet, getting a small drink of water, saying "good night," and going to bed. Signal that bedtime is approaching by keeping lights dim, reducing noise, and moving activities closer to the bedroom.

- Select a bedtime based on when your child naturally gets sleepy. If your child routinely falls asleep at a certain time, it's best to have them get into bed at around that time. This helps avoid long periods of lying awake in bed.

Sleep Setting

- The best place for your child to sleep depends on what works for your family and how your home is set up. Whether your child sleeps in their own room or in a shared room, it's important for them to fall asleep where you want them to sleep the rest of the night. And, if possible, have your child sleep in their own bed, alone.

- Conditions that tend to promote sleep are a cool room temperature, comfortable bedding, quiet surroundings (or steady background noise like a fan or white noise machine), and as little light as possible (a dim nightlight or a hallway light may be needed for children who fear the dark). Any objects in the room or on the bed should be ones that promote comfort and sleep. If possible, remove any objects that might encourage your child to be awake and active at night.

During the Night

- Being able to fall asleep on one's own is an important skill that all children need to learn. If your child needs a lot of support to fall asleep, like being rocked or held, having someone lie in bed with them, being driven around in a car, or other strategies that rely on you or another caregiver, try fading this over time so that your child can learn to fall asleep on their own. The idea behind fading support is essentially to do a little less each time. For example, if you're lying in bed with your child, try sitting at the edge of the bed instead. If you're sitting on the edge of the bed, try sitting on the floor or just outside the bedroom door. If your child is hugging your entire body as they fall asleep, try giving them just your hand to hold or a pillow to hug instead. The goal is for you to be able to leave the room while your child is still awake, so they can fall asleep alone.

- If your child can fall asleep without you present, they'll be much more likely to go back to sleep on their own if they wake up during the night. Waking up briefly during the night is a natural part of sleep. Most of us go right back to sleep. This is a skill you can teach your child. Many children have a habit of looking for a parent when they wake up at night. A good way to help your child stay in their own bed at night is to show them what you'd like to happen by creating a story. The story should have your child as the main character and describe how they carry through with a sequence of actions. (See the "Example of a Sleep Story" below.)

- Other strategies you can try include using a clock that lights up at a certain time in the morning and teaching your child to stay in bed until the light goes on, or sleeping on a mattress outside your child's bedroom door for a few nights so that if they try to come out, you can tell them to go back to bed. As your child is learning to sleep on their own through the night, keep any interactions as short and uninteresting as possible. Keep your voice soft and avoid anything that might stimulate your child and make it harder for them to go back to sleep. This is one of the few times in life when it helps to be as dull and boring as possible.

- Ensuring safety during the night sometimes requires a way to monitor your child's room by video, a way to hear if your child leaves their room at night, and a way to secure any dangerous items in the house and any exits from the house. Some children sleep well in a safety bed that has a zipper enclosure to keep them from leaving their bed at night.

If putting in place a sleep improvement plan feels daunting, pick just one action that feels the easiest and give it a try.

Example of a Sleep Story

During the day I like to spend time outside. (Insert a photo of your child outdoors.)

I also like to _____. (Insert examples of physical activities your child enjoys and photos of your child engaged in these physical activities.)

When I spend time outdoors and when I'm active during the day, I sleep better at night.

At _____ o'clock I start getting ready for bed. First, I take a bath. (Insert a photo of bath time.)

Next, I put on my pajamas. (Insert a photo of your child putting on pajamas.)

Then I brush my teeth. (Insert a photo of your child brushing their teeth.)

When I go back to my bedroom, I can pick a story to read with Mom or Dad. (Insert a photo of you and your child reading a book together in their room.)

After we read the book, we turn off the lights and I get into bed. My parents leave the room. I lie in bed with my eyes closed, breathe slowly, and relax my body. I can sleep with my favorite stuffed animal and my special blanket. (Insert a photo of your child sleeping in bed with their preferred sleep items.)

If I wake up at night, I stay in my bed and stay quiet until I fall back asleep. When my mom or dad comes into my room in the morning, I get out of bed and start my day. (Insert a photo of your child getting out of bed in the morning.)

Abby, a six-year-old nonspeaking girl with autism, routinely woke up after four hours of sleep and would be wide awake for several hours. She would leave her room, turn on lights, run around the house, and wake up her sisters and parents. To keep her from doing this, her parents took turns sleeping in the same room with her.

As part of my evaluation, I learned that Abby was getting a lot of exercise and sunlight during the day, had a good bedtime routine, and didn't have any signs of co-occurring medical conditions that would interfere with sleep. So I felt that what she needed was to learn how to go back to sleep when she woke up at night. I asked her parents not to sleep in Abby's room and instead to put a mattress outside her room where one of them would sleep for the next four nights. Each time Abby got up, they would tell her from outside the room, "Go back to bed." If Abby tried to leave the room, they would bring her back to bed. With the bedroom door slightly open, they could keep an eye on her to make sure she was safe. Before starting this, they were to create a story to explain to Abby what would happen.

For two weeks after, I didn't hear from Abby's parents. Then I got this email, which Abby's dad sent to me and her schoolteacher, behavior therapy supervisor, occupational therapist, and speech-language therapist:

Dear Team Abby,

Over the past few weeks, Abby has been enjoying summer break. She spent time at the beach, Children's Museum, botanical garden, and community swimming pool. But the big news for us is that Abby has learned to sleep! We did Dr. Goh's four-day plan, and really, we saw results after the second day. We started the plan two weeks ago. The spare bed is out of Abby's room, her mom and I sleep in our own room every night, and Abby has had more sleep in the last two weeks than in her whole life. It never occurred to us that Abby had to be taught how to sleep. We're really starting to understand that if we can find the way to teach her, she can learn so much.

Sleep is one of my favorite areas to work on with families because dramatic, unexpected improvements can happen quickly. A child who starts to sleep well is like a new child, and this gives everyone else at home a real shot at sleeping well, too.

Support for Improving Sleep

DIETARY CHANGES

Your child's diet can influence the quality of their sleep. There's no single diet that improves sleep for everyone, but we know that a lack of key nutrients, such as magnesium, calcium, iron, and vitamins A, C, D, E, and K, can be associated with sleep problems. We also know that eating foods high in carbohydrates that cause blood sugar level to spike (high glycemic index foods like sugary snacks) are associated with more frequent night wakings and reduced time spent in deep sleep. Caffeine intake can also disrupt sleep. The Mediterranean diet—a diet rich in vegetables, fruits, whole grains, and olive oil, with moderate amounts of fish and low amounts of meat and dairy—has been shown in research studies to improve sleep. If a nutrient deficiency is present, such as iron deficiency, correcting the deficiency through dietary changes or by taking a dietary supplement can improve sleep.

NUTRITIONAL SUPPLEMENTS

A number of nutritional supplements can help promote sleep for some people. Research studies for most of these supplements in autism are limited, and it's important to use these only under the guidance of a qualified health-care professional:

- Melatonin
- Magnesium
- Glycine
- Cannabidiol
- L-tryptophan or 5-hydroxytryptophan
- L-theanine
- Herbal therapies

MEDICATIONS

These are some of the medications used to promote sleep in autism.

- Clonidine (Catapres or Kapvay)
- Trazodone (many brand names)
- Mirtazapine (Remeron)
- Gabapentin (Neurontin)
- Antihistamine medications

NEUROMODULATION THERAPIES
(DEVICE THERAPIES)

Cranial electrotherapy stimulation (CES)

This therapy involves a device that delivers a small electrical current through electrodes placed on the ears. This electrical stimulation influences the activity of nerves, such as the vagus nerve and other cranial nerves. In a research study conducted at Cortica, we found sleep improvement in about a third of children who used CES.

Biofeedback

This therapy uses technology to measure biological activity, like breathing, heart rate, sweat gland activity, muscle contraction, temperature, or brain electrical activity. A person is then taught strategies to alter their own biological activity, like relaxing certain muscles or thinking certain thoughts, or they receive other forms of feedback that help shift biological activity. Biofeedback is a category of therapy that includes many possible devices and approaches that all use some form of technology to help teach new ways to regulate your body.

GASTROINTESTINAL CONDITIONS

The gastrointestinal (GI) tract runs from the mouth to the anus and includes the throat, esophagus (the tube that connects the throat to the stomach), stomach, and intestines. Until recently, most doctors didn't give much thought to how the GI tract affects the brain. But research now shows that the brain and GI tract influence each other in powerful ways. The most direct connection is through nerves that run between the brain and GI tract. In fact, the GI tract has its own complex web of neurons, called the *enteric nervous system*, that's nicknamed the "second brain." These neurons control activities of the GI tract, such as the wavelike movements that push food forward. They send information like pain signals back to the brain when there's too much gas or stool causing the walls of the gut to stretch. The GI tract also influences the brain by producing hormones that travel to the brain sending signals of hunger or fullness. The health of the GI tract and the bacteria and other microorganisms that live there (called the microbiota) determine what's absorbed from the GI tract into the bloodstream. Once in the bloodstream, substances can travel to the brain and influence how it functions. All the channels of direct and indirect communication between the GI tract and the brain are now collectively called the *gut-brain axis*.

Research in this area has taken off in recent years, including over a thousand research studies looking at the GI tract and autism. Researchers have made several important findings. First, GI symptoms, like constipation, diarrhea, abdominal pain, reflux, and feeding difficulties, together affect close to 80 percent of autistic children. So it's important to recognize the signs that these are occurring and know the steps that can help. Second, GI symptoms are more likely for children who also have other co-occurring conditions, such as epilepsy, sleep disturbance, or mental health symptoms, especially anxiety. Third, GI symptoms can trigger other changes, like an increase in repetitive behaviors, a decrease in social interaction, trouble focusing, difficulty sleeping, hyperactivity, irritability, and even aggressive or self-injurious behaviors. Any worrisome behaviors or changes should prompt a thorough search for GI symptoms.

Our understanding of GI health in autism has come a long way, but there's still a lot we don't know. One of the big questions has to do with what comes first, the features of autism or the GI issues—the chicken or the egg. For example, some research studies have found that autistic children have different gut microbiota (bacteria and other microorganisms) than neurotypical children. It's possible that the sensory processing differences and reduced behavioral flexibility that are part of autism lead to food selectivity and a restricted diet, which changes the microbiota. We know that what we eat has a major effect on our gut microbiota. But it's also possible that poor gut health and altered microbiota lead to changes in the chemicals within the GI tract, which are then absorbed into the bloodstream, travel to the brain, and alter the chemical and electrical function of the brain in ways that increase autistic features. We know that microbiota can influence how a person thinks, feels, and behaves. Some studies have even shown that changing the microbiota by introducing certain probiotics or other treatments can improve gut health and reduce autistic features. As more research studies are done to shed light on these questions, it's very likely we'll find that the role of microbiota is different for different children, which is why some may respond to interventions targeting gut function and others may not.

With many questions still unanswered, what can you do for your child? First, it's important to recognize signs that your child may have abdominal pain or discomfort. Some children can describe what they're feeling, but others may show indirect signs, like pushing their abdomen onto objects, chewing non-edible objects, or constantly eating or drinking. Some children have an increase in irritability, aggression, self-injury, unusual vocalizations (like frequent swallowing or moaning), repeated movements (like grimacing or tapping), hyperactivity, difficulty sleeping, or increased anxiety.

In addition to recognizing potential signs of abdominal discomfort, you can learn about common GI conditions in autism and how to treat them.

Constipation is generally defined as fewer than three bowel movements per week, but children who have bowel movements more often may still be constipated. Signs of constipation include hard poop, difficulty with bowel movements, a small amount of poop with each bowel movement, and smelly gas. Children are more likely to be constipated if they have low fiber in the diet, low fluid intake, reduced awareness of internal body sensations, heightened stress, rigid behaviors, or a history of uncomfortable bowel movements, which can lead to fear and avoidance of having bowel movements. One or two soft, formed bowel movements of moderate to large volume most days of the week is the goal for most children. Steps that can help reach this goal include increasing fiber and water intake, encouraging physical activity, and taking steps to reduce anxiety and stress. Supplements containing fiber, magnesium, probiotics, prebiotics, and many others are widely available and can help with constipation. Medications for constipation are also available over-the-counter or with a prescription.

Diarrhea is loose, watery bowel movements several times a day. Diarrhea can be caused by infections, food allergies and intolerances, certain medications, or other problems of the GI tract, like inflammatory conditions or bacterial overgrowth. Constipation is more common than diarrhea in autistic children, but some children have a pattern of alternating diarrhea and constipation. Sometimes this is caused by leakage of diarrhea around hard stool that's blocking the bowel. Diarrhea can come with abdominal cramping, pain, or nausea. If your child has diarrhea that lasts longer than a week or comes and goes on a regular basis, it's important to seek a thorough evaluation with a medical provider who's knowledgeable about GI conditions in autism.

Reflux (also called gastroesophageal reflux disease) occurs when acid from the stomach flows backward into the esophagus. This backwash, called acid reflux, can cause pain in the chest or abdomen, a burning sensation in the chest (heartburn), food or sour liquid in the throat or mouth, the sensation of a lump in the throat, or trouble swallowing. For some people, acid reflux can cause a cough, laryngitis, or asthma. Reflux is more likely when lying down and after a large meal, especially a meal high in fat. Some autistic children are predisposed to reflux. This could be for a variety of reasons: the ring of muscle (called a sphincter) that usually blocks acid from flowing from the stomach up into the esophagus may be loose; the movement of food through the GI tract may be delayed; or the types or amounts of food the child eats could worsen reflux. Because reflux comes and goes, it can cause intermittent pain. Pain can become more constant if acid reflux happens frequently enough to cause inflammation of the esophagus (called esophagitis). Understandably, this kind of pain can lead to irritability and behavioral outbursts. Dietary changes and medications for reflux can be very effective. Since medical testing for reflux usually requires an invasive procedure, a common approach doctors use when there's concern for reflux is to bypass the procedure and start a medication to see if symptoms improve.

Feeding problems, like food aversions and a limited diet, are also considered conditions of the GI system. Depending on the type and degree of feeding problems, they can also alter the microbiota and contribute to constipation, diarrhea, reflux, and other medical conditions. The best approach is a comprehensive nutrition and feeding evaluation and a therapy program that takes into account all the different factors that influence what a child eats (like sensory, motor, social, behavioral, and medical factors).

Other GI conditions can also occur, like celiac disease, food allergies and intolerances, eosinophilic esophagitis, other inflammatory GI conditions, and small intestine bacterial overgrowth. Research studies have found celiac disease to be more common in autism and are investigating whether this may also be true of other inflammatory and infectious GI conditions. Since it's possible for an autistic child to have any of these GI conditions, it's important to work with a doctor who can gather appropriate information and conduct any needed tests.

MITOCHONDRIAL DISEASE AND DYSFUNCTION

Mitochondria have been in the spotlight in recent years because of their role in virtually every chronic health condition. These tiny structures inside of cells convert nutrients from the food we eat into energy. Mitochondria are called the "powerhouse" of the cell because they provide energy for all the body's functions. But mitochondria do far more than generate fuel for the body. They're also involved in many other complex biochemical functions within cells, so when they aren't working properly, many different symptoms can appear.

A small percentage (less than 5 percent) of autistic children are diagnosed with a mitochondrial disease. These diseases fall within the category of metabolic disorders with a genetic cause that we discussed earlier in this chapter. Signs of mitochondrial disease in an autistic child often include low energy (getting tired easily), GI symptoms, developmental regression, epilepsy, hormone abnormalities, and problems with motor function, including weakness, incoordination, or movement disorders. Genetic testing for these conditions should include whole exome sequencing and mitochondrial DNA sequencing. Laboratory tests should include a broad panel of tests on blood and urine to look for indicators of mitochondrial disease. Depending on the specific type of mitochondrial disease, supplementing the diet with a particular vitamin, mineral, or other nutritional supplement may improve symptoms.

A much larger proportion of autistic children—as many as 80 percent—have a milder condition called mitochondrial dysfunction. *Mitochondrial dysfunction* is a broad term that includes many different ways that mitochondria may not be functioning optimally. For example, *mitochondrial dysfunction* can refer to underactivity of mitochondria (deficiency) as well as overactivity. Signs of mitochondrial dysfunction overlap with those seen in mitochondrial disease, but may be different depending on the type and degree of mitochondrial dysfunction. Diagnostic and treatment approaches also overlap with those for mitochondrial disease. Research on the nuances of mitochondrial dysfunction in autism continues to advance and will likely bring new therapies in the future.

· ·

Mitochondrial Support

LIFESTYLE CHANGES

Good quality sleep and regular exercise benefit mitochondrial function. Situations that increase stress on the body, like illness, dehydration, fever, extreme temperatures, surgery, anesthesia, prolonged fasting, and sleep deprivation, can disrupt mitochondrial function, especially if they occur at the same time. Certain medications may affect mitochondrial function, and some pesticides and other chemicals common in the environment may, too. If your child has mitochondrial disease or dysfunction, talk with your doctor about how to manage these potential stressors.

DIETARY CHANGES

Dietary approaches to support mitochondrial function depend on the type of mitochondrial disease or dysfunction that's present. There's no single diet that's best for everyone.

NUTRITIONAL SUPPLEMENTS

A number of nutritional supplements are used to support mitochondrial function. Use these only under the guidance of a qualified health-care professional:

- L-carnitine
- Coenzyme Q10
- Vitamin C
- Vitamin E

- B vitamins
- Creatine
- Alpha-lipoic acid
- L-arginine
- N-acetylcysteine (NAC)
- Other nutrients, many with antioxidant properties

OTHER

Since chronic stress can impair mitochondrial function, any intervention that helps reduce chronic stress, including device therapies and developmental-behavioral approaches, has the potential to benefit mitochondrial function.

AUTONOMIC NERVOUS SYSTEM DYSFUNCTION

Many people are familiar with the general makeup of the body's nervous system, which includes the brain, spinal cord, and nerves that the brain and spinal cord send out to the rest of the body. But fewer people are aware of the *autonomic* nervous system, which is the part of the nervous system that regulates our internal organs, like our heart, lungs, and digestive system, and does this automatically without our conscious control (the words *autonomic* and *automatic* have similar meaning). Our heart rate, breathing, and food digestion are just a few examples of functions controlled by the autonomic nervous system. Luckily, we don't have to think about these activities—they happen on their own.

Like any other part of the human body, the autonomic nervous system sometimes doesn't function well. In autism the trouble is usually with the balance between the two branches of the autonomic nervous system: *sympathetic* and *parasympathetic*. Nerves of the sympathetic branch reach many organs and stimulate them at the same time (*sympathetic* means "to feel together"). The parasympathetic branch works alongside the sympathetic branch to produce opposite and complementary effects. For example, when sympathetic nerves are stimulated, they cause an increase in heart rate, stronger heart contractions, faster breathing, increased adrenaline, and the release of stored sugar to be used as energy. All of these prepare the body to respond to stressful situations with a "fight, flight, or freeze" response. The parasympathetic branch, on the other hand, promotes a "rest and digest" response by slowing the heart rate, slowing breathing, reducing adrenaline, and allowing the digestive system to move food forward and to have a bowel movement. Stimulation of organs by both these branches occurs at the same time, and it's this delicate and shifting balance that allows us to adapt to changing circumstances.

For many autistic people there's an imbalance—an overactive sympathetic branch, an underactive parasympathetic branch, or both. This means the body is in a state of stress more often than it should be. This is described as a state of *hyper-arousal*. For a smaller number the imbalance is in the opposite direction, called *hypo-arousal*, and they might have trouble adapting to environments where greater energy and faster responses are needed. Some autistic people fluctuate between these states. We don't know all the reasons for autonomic imbalance, but one likely reason has to do with how the autistic brain processes sensory information. For those who tend toward a state of hyper-arousal, there's often an accompanying over-responsiveness to sensory stimuli, and many settings may feel overstimulating, unpredictable, and stressful. The demands of communicating and interacting socially in many settings may also add to stress. We know that living in a world designed by neurotypical minds can be stressful for someone with a neurodivergent mind.

To precisely measure a person's sympathetic and parasympathetic nervous system function on a continuous basis requires specialized equipment and software. More researchers are looking at how common devices, like watches and other wearables, can be used to track heart rate and other body functions to learn more about a person's autonomic nervous system. Even without these objective measures, we can learn a lot by observing a child's behavior, level of energy and activity, and even their pattern of bowel movements. If there are signs of imbalance in the autonomic nervous system, a doctor can recommend certain medications and other treatments to reduce sympathetic overactivity or stimulate parasympathetic activity.

Support for the Autonomic Nervous System

LIFESTYLE CHANGES

Any changes to routines or activities that reduce stress and promote calm can help the function of the autonomic nervous system. Proactively offering your child information so they know what to expect is one of the most effective strategies. Frequent opportunities for exercise and outdoor activities can also be beneficial.

DIETARY CHANGES

Try to reduce foods that cause blood sugar to spike, like sugary snacks, baked goods, and other simple carbohydrates.

NUTRITIONAL SUPPLEMENTS

Many nutritional supplements have the potential to promote a state of relaxation. Use these only under the guidance of a qualified health-care professional: vitamin B6, L-theanine, glycine, magnesium, and herbal therapies.

MEDICATIONS

Beta-adrenergic blocking medications (also known as beta-blockers)

These medications work by blocking the effects of the hormone epinephrine (adrenaline). They are often used to treat high blood pressure, migraine headaches, anxiety, and heart conditions. Research studies of autism have found that the beta-blocker propranolol can sometimes improve behavior, anxiety, and cognitive function.

Alpha-2 adrenergic agonists: clonidine (Catapres or Kapvay) and guanfacine (Tenex or Intuniv)

These are medications that counter the activity of the sympathetic nervous system. Research studies have found that these medications can improve attention, hyperactivity, and impulsivity in autistic children.

NEUROMODULATION THERAPIES (DEVICE THERAPIES)

Cranial electrotherapy stimulation (CES)

This therapy involves use of a device that delivers a small electrical current through electrodes placed on the ears. The electrical stimulation influences the activity of nerves, including the vagus nerve, which increases the activity of the parasympathetic nervous system. In a study conducted at Cortica, autistic children receiving CES showed improvements in anxiety and emotion dysregulation.

Biofeedback

This therapy uses technology to measure biological activity, like breathing, heart rate, sweat gland activity, muscle contraction, temperature, or the brain's electrical activity. A person is then taught strategies to alter their own biological activity, like relaxing certain muscles or thinking certain thoughts, or they receive other forms of feedback that help reduce the body's stress response and promote a "rest-and-digest" state.

- Therapies that build skills in sensory processing and motor function, like occupational therapy, physical therapy, music therapy, behavior therapy, and many others
- Counseling and other therapies that teach stress-reduction techniques and emotion regulation

IMMUNE SYSTEM

An autistic child may have allergies, autoimmune conditions, or immune deficiencies just as any other child might. But differences in sensory processing, communication, and behavior can make it harder to detect the signs, so it may take more attention and support to properly assess and treat these conditions.

Researchers are actively investigating alterations in the immune system in autism and have found atypical activation of some elements of the immune system. The immune system is highly complex, so it's still too soon to know what steps should be taken based on these research findings. But we know that allergies, autoimmune conditions, and immune deficiencies can occur in autistic children, and we should do appropriate tests if signs of these conditions appear. It's also important to keep in mind that nutrition, exercise, and stress-reduction have well-proven benefits for the immune system, and any improvements you make in these areas are likely to have lasting benefits for your child's health. You'll learn more about this in chapter 6.

Diagnosing and Treating
Co-occurring Mental Health Conditions

If an autistic child has a hard time focusing, worries a great deal, has persistent disturbing thoughts (obsessions), or has a depressed mood, these may be signs of a co-occurring mental health condition. In the past these were often overlooked—sometimes brushed off as "part of autism." But not all autistic children experience these symptoms. When they do, it's important to identify them and provide appropriate care, just as we should for any person.

Overall, mental health diagnoses are thought to be about twice as common in autism, and these can potentially affect a child's quality of life even more than the core features of autism or co-occurring medical conditions. These diagnoses are made on the basis of how a child is feeling, thinking, and behaving, so it's important to give children the opportunity to share their thoughts and emotions using whatever mode of communication works best for them. Identifying these conditions is essential to providing quality care.

ATTENTION-DEFICIT/HYPERACTIVITY DISORDER (ADHD)

Hyperactivity and difficulty focusing are the hallmark features of ADHD. Difficulty focusing can occur during routine activities, like schoolwork, chores, or play, and may cause a child to be easily distracted and appear forgetful. Hyperactivity can mean having trouble staying seated and appearing constantly "on the go." Children may fidget or squirm, and some may run or climb in settings that aren't meant for this. Hyperactivity can also appear as impulsive behavior, in which a child has difficulty waiting their turn, interrupts others, takes over what others are doing, or moves in fast and unpredictable ways. Many of these behaviors are common for toddlers, but for older children these behaviors can get in the way of social relationships or school performance, so an ADHD diagnosis may be appropriate. ADHD also means challenges with executive functions like organizing, managing time efficiently, prioritizing tasks, and making decisions.

There are three types of ADHD: inattentive, hyperactive/impulsive, and combined. To make a diagnosis, a physician or psychologist will interview caregivers and may also ask for standardized questionnaires to be completed. Computer-based tests to measure attention and impulsivity are also available and can help with diagnosis. Sometimes ADHD symptoms have an underlying medical cause. For example, seizures can cause periods of inattention and difficulty focusing, and research studies have found that up to a quarter of children with ADHD have abnormal electrical activity in the brain that indicates they are more prone to having seizures. Another medical condition that can contribute to difficulty focusing is iron deficiency. If this is detected through blood testing, supplementing your child's diet with iron may improve ADHD symptoms. Inadequate sleep, anxiety, GI conditions, and sensory processing difficulties can all contribute to inattention or hyperactivity and should also be considered when determining the best approach to treatment.

Medications are often used for ADHD, but there are other important steps to take first. ADHD symptoms can improve when children are given plenty of opportunities for physical activity during the day. Reducing time spent on electronic devices can also help. At school, many children with ADHD benefit from sitting near the teacher and away from doors, windows, and other distractions. Other useful strategies include taking breaks that involve movement activities, using fidget toys, having extra time to complete assignments, and engaging in rewarding experiences right after completing tasks. You can also write down instructions and other important information where your child can easily find them. Some research studies have found that children benefit from changes to their diet, like reducing sugar and highly processed foods, especially those with artificial colorings, preservatives, and other additives. Other studies have found that omega-3 fatty acids (found in fish oil and other foods and supplements) may help ADHD symptoms, and for children with iron deficiency, it's important to increase iron intake in the diet or take an iron supplement.

Medications for ADHD fall into two categories—stimulants and non-stimulants—and research studies have found that both classes can help with ADHD symptoms in autistic children. Recently, the FDA approved a software "brain training" program called EndeavorRx to treat ADHD symptoms that looks and feels like a video game. Because there are so many potential components to an effective approach to ADHD, it's important to work closely with your child's doctor. With your knowledge of your child, and your doctor's expertise, you'll be able to co-create an effective, multifaceted treatment plan.

Support for ADHD

LIFESTYLE CHANGES

Increasing physical activity

Reducing time on electronic devices

School accommodations, like sitting near the teacher and away from doors, windows, and other distractions; taking breaks that involve movement activities; using fidget toys; having extra time to complete assignments; providing rewarding experiences immediately following task completion; and writing down instructions and other important information where your child can easily reference it.

DIETARY CHANGES

Reducing sugar and highly processed foods, especially those with artificial colorings, preservatives, and other additives, may benefit some children.

NUTRITIONAL SUPPLEMENTS

For children with iron deficiency, increasing intake of iron in the diet or taking an iron supplement may help.

Omega-3 fatty acids may have the potential to help some children.

MEDICATIONS

Many medications are available for ADHD and come in a variety of forms, including liquids, tablets, capsules, patches, and chewable tablets. They also come in short-acting, long-acting, immediate-release, and delayed-release forms. Children sometimes need to try several medications to determine the best option for them. Some doctors use pharmacogenetic (or pharmacogenomic) testing to help guide the selection of medications. Although physicians and researchers don't all agree on whether this type of testing has benefits, many physicians find this test helpful, and the cost may be covered in part by your insurance.

Non-stimulants
Alpha-2 adrenergic agonists: clonidine (Catapres and Kapvay) and guanfacine (Tenex and Intuniv)

Medications that influence activity of the neurotransmitter norepinephrine: atomoxetine (Strattera) and viloxazine (Qelbree)

These medications influence activity of the neurotransmitters norepinephrine and dopamine and also have other effects on the brain and body. These medications stimulate the sympathetic nervous system.

Methylphenidate—ADHD medications with methylphenidate are known by the brand names Ritalin, Concerta, Metadate, Methylin, Aptensio, Focalin, Quillivant, Cotempla, and others.

Amphetamines—ADHD medications with amphetamines are known by the brand names Adderall, Vyvanse, Dexedrine, Dyanavel, ProCentra, Evekeo, and others.

NEUROMODULATION THERAPIES (DEVICE THERAPIES)

EndeavorRx is a software "brain training" program that looks and feels like a video game.

Other device-based therapeutics for ADHD appear promising but still have limited research to support their use, such as trigeminal nerve stimulation (TNS) and EEG neurofeedback.

DEVELOPMENTAL AND BEHAVIORAL APPROACHES

Therapies that help with sensory processing, motor function, and social-emotional abilities can help children with ADHD. Occupational therapy, physical therapy, music therapy, behavior therapy, counseling, and many other developmental-behavioral approaches all have potential benefits.

ANXIETY

All people experience worries and fears, but when they get in the way of everyday activities, we consider them symptoms of anxiety.

Unpleasant physical sensations, like shortness of breath, a racing heart, or a general feeling of discomfort and unease in the body, are common signs of anxiety and are related to overactivity of the sympathetic nervous system. Many autistic children experience anxiety, possibly because of sensory processing differences that make environments less comfortable and less predictable and social difficulties that make it harder to predict and adapt to other people. Some children describe feeling anxious, nervous, worried, or fearful. Other children may show their anxiety by increasing repetitive behaviors like counting, lining up objects, and repetitive movements or vocalizations. For some children, anxiety increases with changes in routine, social interactions, new people, new settings, or being faced with difficult tasks.

Obsessive-compulsive disorder (OCD) is characterized by unwanted and repeated thoughts (obsessions). To get relief from these thoughts, a person with OCD may engage in certain repeated behaviors (compulsions). Engaging in repeated behaviors—such as putting things in a certain order, counting, tapping, or touching—is also part of autism, but this is usually done as a way to receive sensory input and engage with the environment. When these actions are done to reduce unwanted thoughts, they're classified as compulsions, and may be considered obsessive-compulsive symptoms rather than autistic features. It's not always possible to tell what's motivating the behaviors and whether they represent autistic features or symptoms of OCD.

By keeping in mind that your child may be experiencing anxiety, you're more likely to see opportunities to provide positive messages and reassurance to help reduce worries and fears. Offering information to help your child know what to expect from new experiences can go a long way to making those experiences less stressful. As autistic actor Mickey Rowe says, "There is a perception of autistic people that we don't do well with change, but I prefer to reframe it as we do well when we know what to expect." Professional services, like counseling and occupational therapy, can help your child and family members learn strategies for reducing anxiety. Changes to the diet may be helpful since certain foods, like refined sugars and caffeine, can make anxiety worse. Certain medications, like stimulants, can also increase anxiety, and this is important to keep in mind for children taking stimulant therapy for ADHD who may also have anxiety. Many nutritional supplements, medications, and other therapies can also help reduce anxiety.

Support for Anxiety

LIFESTYLE CHANGES

Provide positive messages and reassurance to help reduce worries and fears. Offering information to help your child know what to expect from new experiences can go a long way toward making those experiences less stressful and more enjoyable.

DIETARY CHANGES

Reduce intake of caffeine and processed foods with refined sugars.

NUTRITIONAL SUPPLEMENTS

Many nutritional supplements have the potential to promote relaxation and reduce anxiety, but research studies are limited. Use these only under the guidance of a qualified health-care professional: vitamin B6, L-theanine, glycine, magnesium, cannabidiol, N-acetylcysteine, vitamin B9 (folate, best used in the form of L-methylfolate or folinic acid), and herbal therapies.

Medications that influence neurotransmitter function in the brain:

- Medications that act mainly on the neurotransmitter serotonin: citalopram (Celexa), escitalopram (Lexapro), fluoxetine (Prozac), paroxetine (Paxil), sertraline (Zoloft), and others.
- Medications that act on serotonin and norepinephrine: duloxetine (Cymbalta), venlafaxine (Effexor), desvenlafaxine (Pristiq), and others.
- Medications that influence the activity of the neurotransmitter gamma-aminobutyric acid (GABA): clonazepam (Klonopin), lorazepam (Ativan), diazepam (Valium), and others.

Medications that act on the sympathetic nervous system:

- Beta-blockers and alpha-2 adrenergic agonists (see the section on supporting the function of the autonomic nervous system for more information).

NEUROMODULATION THERAPIES (DEVICE THERAPIES)

Therapies that help balance the function of the autonomic nervous system can also help anxiety. These include cranial electrotherapy stimulation (CES) and biofeedback (see the section on supporting the function of the autonomic nervous system for more information).

Transcranial magnetic stimulation (TMS) uses machine-generated magnetic fields to stimulate electrical activity in specific brain areas. TMS is mainly used to treat depression but is sometimes used to treat obsessive-compulsive disorder (OCD).

Counseling, occupational therapy, and many other approaches can help teach emotion regulation.

DEPRESSION

Feelings of sadness, hopelessness, low self-esteem, and not fitting in are increasingly common in our society, and research studies indicate that depression is more common in autism. So it's important to look for signs of depression in autistic children, teens, and adults, especially in those who may not be able to express their feelings clearly. Signs of depression may include sleeping too little or too much, low energy, irritability, reduced enjoyment in activities, difficulty concentrating, anxiety, and changes in appetite. Many effective treatments for depression are available and overlap a great deal with treatments for anxiety.

GENDER INCONGRUENCE

Gender incongruence is defined as a condition where a person's sense of gender identity doesn't match the gender assigned to them at birth. For example, a person assigned a gender of male at birth may later identify as female or nonbinary. Research studies have shown that gender incongruence is more common in autism and could potentially lead to distress or difficulties in a person's social life, work life, or other important areas (called *gender dysphoria*). There's a lot we're still learning about gender identity and autism, but by keeping in mind that your child might experience their gender identity in unique ways, you'll be better equipped to find ways to support them.

Diagnosing and Treating Co-occurring Developmental or Behavioral Conditions

Conditions that co-occur with autism can be grouped into the categories of medical, mental health, developmental, and behavioral, as you've seen in this chapter, but these categories are overlapping and the boundaries between them are not as clear as the categories suggest. Although we think of certain brain functions as part of mental health and others as part of child development or behavior, they all reside in the brain. Still, these categories are helpful when thinking about autism's co-occurring conditions. They help us make sure we aren't neglecting an area of your child's health or development that could improve with support.

SENSORY PROCESSING DISORDER/DIFFERENCES (SPD)

After decades of research showing that differences in sensory processing are central to autism, these features became part of autism diagnostic criteria in 2013. Because differences in sensory processing are among autism's core features, professionals generally don't make a separate diagnosis of SPD if a child already has an autism diagnosis.

DEVELOPMENTAL COORDINATION DISORDER (DCD) OR DEVELOPMENTAL DYSPRAXIA

Children who have difficulty coordinating movements may be diagnosed with DCD or dyspraxia (the terms are interchangeable). A child might have trouble with accuracy, speed, and coordination when performing motor skills, which can make it harder to carry out essential daily routines.

Because DCD is so common in autism, and because motor skills affect all aspects of behavior, some researchers believe that motor differences should be considered a core feature of autism. I agree with them and hope that one day the accurate measurement of movement differences in autism will have a place in autism diagnosis.

Children with autism and DCD can benefit from occupational therapy, physical therapy, music therapy, dance/movement therapy, and many other therapies, as well as sports, music, and recreational activities that build sensory and motor skills.

CONDITIONS RELATED TO COGNITIVE OR INTELLECTUAL FUNCTION

As we discussed in chapter 4, cognitive and intellectual abilities span a broad range of mental abilities, including a range of skills related to attention, memory, language, and information processing. Most physicians and psychologists who specialize in neurodevelopment find it more helpful to focus on each of these cognitive functions on their own rather than grouping them together. For example, a child with difficulty focusing may have ADHD and may benefit from the many therapies available for ADHD. A child with a speech-language delay will benefit from speech-language therapy. These diagnoses help highlight precise areas where a child can benefit from support. Broader diagnoses, on the other hand, like cognitive impairment or intellectual disability, lack this level of specificity.

Children who have difficulty learning foundational academic skills for reading, writing, or math during the first years of school may be diagnosed with a specific learning disorder or developmental learning disorder. These diagnoses generally aren't given if a child already has an autism diagnosis. As we know, autism comes with a unique cognitive style that can make conforming with neurotypical academic standards challenging. So an autistic child may be able to acquire skills in these areas in different ways than how they're taught in a standard school curriculum. For this reason, these diagnoses have less of a role for most autistic children.

LANGUAGE

Difficulty using language for social interaction is a core feature of autism and is referred to as difficulty with *social pragmatics*. Other language difficulties can also be present for some autistic children. A language disorder diagnosis may be appropriate if a child has difficulty understanding or producing language. Some autistic children also have a condition called childhood apraxia of speech, which involves difficulty making the coordinated movements of the mouth, tongue, lips, and palate needed for speech. Speech-language therapy and other developmental-behavioral approaches that build sensory and motor skills, like occupational therapy and music therapy, can benefit language development. Some research studies have found that folinic acid (vitamin B9) may improve speech for some autistic children.

EMOTION

Difficulty identifying, describing, and expressing emotions is not a core feature of autism but rather a co-occurring condition called *alexithymia* that occurs in about 50 percent of autistic people. Counseling and other therapies that support understanding and expressing emotions can help build skills in this area.

Difficulty regulating emotions (or emotional dysregulation) is another characteristic that can co-occur with autism, but one that's not considered a diagnosis on its own. Emotional dysregulation can lead to behaviors such as aggression, self-injury, tantrums, or meltdowns. *Irritability* is a term that's been used to describe a state of reduced control over one's temper and excessive responses to stimuli. Emotional dysregulation and irritability are similar concepts, and therapies that address any of autism's co-occurring medical, mental health, or developmental conditions have the potential to help. Counseling and many developmental-behavioral approaches, like occupational therapy and music therapy, can teach skills for emotion regulation. Two medications that have been shown in research studies to help with irritability are aripiprazole (Abilify) and risperidone (Risperdal). Like other medications, these have the potential for side effects, but they can be used safely and effectively under the guidance of a qualified physician.

TAKE-HOME MESSAGE

About 50 percent of autistic children have four or more co-occurring diagnoses. A clear understanding of your child's co-occurring diagnoses allows your child to access greater resources and receive better support. Having a complete view of your child's brain and body health is positive, even though it may feel overwhelming at first. Remember that your child hasn't changed from the moment before the diagnosis to the moment of the diagnosis. What's changed for the better is your power to help them.

Addressing autism's co-occurring conditions sets the stage for success in supporting the development of new brain networks. In the next chapter you'll learn more steps for optimizing health to support brain network development "from the inside" through nutrition, exercise, and stress reduction. You'll also learn how to support brain network development "from the outside" by creating learning opportunities at home and selecting professional therapy services.

Chapter 6

A DEVELOPMENTAL SYMPHONY

Composing Brain Networks

Human atoms are the notes, their life the symphony.

—Kyle Hill, science writer and educator

When Max Park was five years old, he touched a Rubik's cube for the first time. Diagnosed with moderate to severe autism at age two, he had difficulty coordinating his hand movements, and his parents thought a Rubik's cube might help his motor development. Imagine their surprise when he began to solve the cube at lightning speed—performing intricate hand sequences and recalling complex formulas from memory. At age fifteen Max set his first of many world records in the competitive sport of speedcubing. The documentary film *The Speed Cubers* shows how this skill created opportunities for Max to expand his communication, form friendships, and handle intense emotions during high-stakes competitions. His remarkable journey is an example of what's possible during the course of childhood brain development in autism.

Brain development, or *neurodevelopment*, refers to the changes in the brain that make it possible to gain new abilities. Neurodevelopment spans six domains you've already been learning about:

- Sensory (how we sense the world around us)
- Motor (how we move our body)
- Cognitive (how we think, including attention, memory, planning, and problem-solving)
- Language (how we understand and use words to communicate)
- Social (how we interact with other people)
- Emotional (how we process feelings)

We know from research studies and firsthand accounts that autistic neurodevelopment can differ from neurotypical development in many ways:

- Skills can develop in a different order. For example, neurotypical children usually crawl before they climb, speak before they read, play peekaboo before they play puzzles, and so on. But for autistic children, milestones can happen in a different order.

- Skills like smiling at others, making eye contact, and imitating gestures are considered prerequisites for higher-level neurotypical development, but they may not be essential for autistic children. In fact, requiring these skills of a child may impede learning instead of supporting it.

- The pace of learning may differ. Autistic children have unique individual profiles, and rather than following the pace of neurotypical development, they may have periods of little noticeable change punctuated by leaps in skill. Autistic children may learn new information independently without instruction, like learning to read without explicitly being taught, and their advancements may go unrecognized by others.

- The learning style is more likely to be characterized by deeply exploring one focused topic instead of showing interest in a wide range of subjects. An autistic child's topic of special interest or "enthusiasm" is a route to developing skills in other areas, just as Max's cubing skill paved the way for growth in social and emotional skills.

Recognizing these differences in autistic neurodevelopment will help you as you set out to grow your child's abilities.

Brain Basics

There are two main avenues for supporting your child's neurodevelopment. One is improving conditions in their body to promote brain development—supporting "from the inside." The other is creating learning opportunities that provide the just-right challenge based on your child's unique developmental profile—supporting "from the outside." Here you'll learn how to do both.

A newborn brain has tens of billions of brain cells called *neurons*. Neurons and other types of brain cells are organized into three major structures. The *brainstem*, which is at the bottom of the brain, connects the brain to the spinal cord and plays an important role in basic functions like breathing, heart rate, sleep, and consciousness. The part of the brain called the *cerebellum* is located near the back of the head and influences control of movements, thoughts, and emotions.

The third part of the brain, the *cerebrum*, is the largest part, and it has two sides called the right and left hemispheres. These hemispheres are responsible for managing our senses, emotions, thoughts, movements, and language. Both hemispheres have four different lobes with specialized functions.

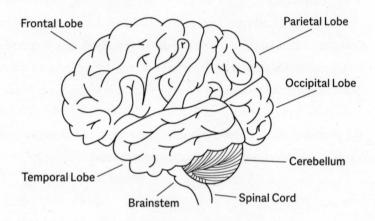

The *frontal lobe* controls voluntary movement, speech production, and "executive" functions like concentration, judgment, self-awareness, reasoning, and problem-solving.

The *parietal lobe* is important for processing sensory information and language.

The *occipital lobe* is the visual processing center of the brain.

The *temporal lobe* interprets sound and has a key role in memory and emotion.

The cerebrum has an outer surface with intricate folds called the *cortex*. This is where most of the information flowing through the nervous system is integrated. Neurons in the cortex send signals through long fibers called *axons* to other parts of the brain.

One of my favorite descriptions of the brain comes from Temple Grandin, who compares it to an office building:

The employees in different parts of the building have their own areas of specialization, but they work together. Some departments work closer together than others. Some departments are more active than others, depending on what the task at hand is. But at the end of the day, they come together to produce a single product: a thought, an action, a response.

Groups of neurons that work together to carry out a specific function—like a thought, action, or response—are called *neural networks*. An exquisite sequence of electrical and chemical events takes place in the brain to create neural networks for new abilities. The chemical events involve molecules called *neurotransmitters*, which are stored inside neurons. When the neurotransmitters are released from the part of the neuron called the *synapse*, they travel to other neurons and stimulate electrical activity. But for that activity to occur, atoms with a positive or negative electrical charge (called *ions*), like sodium, potassium, and chloride, have to move in and out of neurons. These movements take place through *ion channels* in the wall (or *cell membrane*) of the neuron.

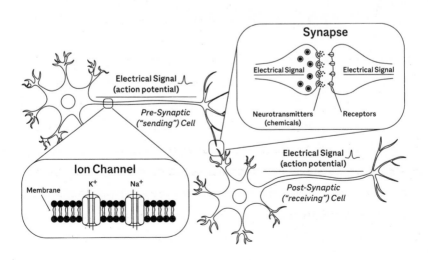

Just like your face is different from everyone else's, your brain is, too. The size and shape of brain structures, the location and pattern of folds in the cortex, and countless other brain features are different from one person to the next. Brains have these differences at birth, influenced by genetics and the prenatal environment, and they become more and more unique over time. Our experiences shape the electrical and chemical activity of the brain, and that changes the physical characteristics of the brain. For example, researchers discovered that London taxi drivers, who learn the names and layout of the city's more than twenty-six thousand streets and thousands of points of interest, have physical changes in a part of the brain called the hippocampus that's important for remembering detailed spatial information. This is just one of countless examples of how experiences—especially those that involve intensive learning—change the physical makeup of the brain.

Brain Differences in Autism

Even before birth, the autistic brain is unique. As a fetus grows, neurons move to particular locations within the brain. In autism these movements are different, so neurons arrive at different destinations. This leads to microscopic changes to brain architecture, especially in the cortex. From about six months to two years of age, the autistic brain grows faster than the neurotypical brain. First, the surface of the cortex grows more quickly, and then the entire brain grows more quickly, so an autistic child's brain is larger early in life, compared with the brains of non-autistic peers. But it doesn't stay that way. By adolescence, there's no longer a difference in brain size. These findings tell us that the autistic brain has its own trajectory, distinct from neurotypical development. Research findings also tell us that the differences exist throughout the brain and span brain networks across all developmental areas.

If we think about the brain as Grandin says, like an office building, then in autism the departments are connected in different ways. This is called altered *connectivity*. Neuroscientists have found that the *prefrontal cortex*—an area that manages cognitive and behavioral flexibility—has fewer connections to other brain regions, and this may explain why thoughts and behaviors tend to be less flexible in autism. Some studies have found more connections between brain areas that are close to each other and fewer connections between brain areas that are farther apart. This could explain the repetitive behaviors and fixed interests in autism, since expanding behaviors and interests relies on complex networks with long-range connections. In a brain imaging study I conducted with colleagues at Columbia University and the University of Southern California, we found that blood flow seems to be greater in areas of the autistic brain where connections are not as strong, which could be a sign that the brain is trying to send more blood to the areas that need more support. In this way and many others, the autistic brain is finding ways to adapt and thrive.

Research studies have also found differences in how neurotransmitters function in autism. Neurons connect with each other by sending neurotransmitters, sometimes called chemical messengers. These messengers move through the small space between neurons called the *synaptic cleft*. Neurotransmitters have wide-ranging effects in the brain, and together they shape a person's thoughts, feelings, and behaviors, much like the ingredients of a recipe come together to create complex flavors. Medications that influence neurotransmitters are among the most common medications used for autism and have the potential to improve how a person thinks, feels, communicates, and behaves.

Dopamine, a neurotransmitter that creates a feeling of reward, may be overactive in some brain regions and underactive in others in autism, and this may vary between people. This could explain why medications that influence dopamine function can sometimes lead to significant improvements in cognition and behavior. Research studies have also looked at the hormone oxytocin, which stimulates the release of dopamine in regions of the brain involved in socialization. Oxytocin exists naturally in the body but can also be delivered as a medication, and some studies have found improvements in social behaviors in autistic people taking oxytocin.

Serotonin is a neurotransmitter that influences many aspects of brain development and brain function. About 98 percent of the body's serotonin is located outside the brain, most of it in the gastrointestinal tract. Researchers are trying to understand how serotonin in the GI tract and in the brain might influence autistic features. Medications that influence serotonin activity are among the most effective for reducing symptoms of anxiety, OCD, and depression.

Gamma-aminobutyric acid (GABA) and glutamate are neurotransmitters that help set a balance between *excitation* (increased activity of neurons) and *inhibition* (reduced activity of neurons). Many research studies have found changes in GABA and glutamate activity in autism, and researchers believe an imbalance between inhibition and excitation may be a key feature of autism.

The brain is an electrical organ, and differences in its electric activity are common in autism. Researchers believe that differences in brain connectivity and neurotransmitter activity set the stage for electrical differences and make seizures and other types of atypical electrical discharges more likely in autism. So differences in electrical activity are not a separate aspect of autism but are closely connected to the differences in brain connectivity and chemistry. Certain dietary changes, nutritional supplements, and medications (reviewed in chapter 5 in the section on epilepsy) can influence the brain's electrical activity and have the potential to improve brain function in autism.

Recently, scientists have also identified important metabolic and immune differences in the autistic brain. In a brain imaging study I conducted with colleagues at Columbia University, we found elevated levels of lactic acid, a sign of altered brain mitochondrial function. In another study we found differences in several compounds in the brain that indicate both altered mitochondrial function and atypical immune system activation. Other studies of metabolism in autism have found reduced folate metabolism and reduced glucose metabolism. New therapies are actively being studied in clinical trials based on these insights into autism biology.

Healthy Body, Healthy Brain

The first and most important step to promote neurodevelopment is one you already know: identifying and treating medical conditions that co-occur with autism. Metabolic disorders, epilepsy, sleep disturbance, gastrointestinal disorders, mitochondrial dysfunction, autonomic nervous system dysfunction, and immune system dysfunction can all interfere with brain development.

Once co-occurring medical conditions are diagnosed and are being treated, you can shift your attention to improving your child's overall health. This means thinking about the food they're eating, their physical activity, the important relationships in their life, and potential sources of stress. Not long ago, most doctors didn't believe that nutrition, exercise, relationships, or stress could make a significant difference for autistic children. But now we know better. Research proves that these have a powerful influence on your child's health and wellness. I've seen remarkable improvements in children's development and behavior with attention to these essential elements of healthy living.

NUTRITION

Two thousand years ago the ancient Greek physician Hippocrates said, "Let food be thy medicine." Modern medical research confirms this historic wisdom: what we eat indeed determines our health. A diet rich in vegetables, fruits, whole grains, and olive oil, with moderate amounts of fish and low amounts of meat and dairy—referred to as the Mediterranean diet—promotes optimal health for most people and is a great starting point for most autistic children.

You've probably heard about dozens of other diets for autism—like gluten-free, casein-free, ketogenic, specific carbohydrate, gut and psychology syndrome (GAPS), and Feingold, along with many others—that involve removing certain foods from the diet. But there are some steps you should take before exploring these for your child. Usually it's helpful to increase the variety of foods your child eats *before* removing foods. Hypersensitivities to the taste, texture, smell, and appearance of food are common in autism. When combined with a tendency for behavioral inflexibility, it makes sense that your child may limit the type and number of foods they're willing to eat. If we remove food from a diet that's already limited, we risk taking away important nutrients.

If your child has difficulty gaining weight, expanding their diet can help them to gain weight and to grow. If your child would benefit by losing weight, then the focus should be on including more foods that are rich in nutrients and lower in calories, instead of highly processed foods that tend to be low in nutrients and high in calories.

Common processed foods	Whole-food alternatives
Salty snacks (potato chips, crackers, etc.)	Nuts, vegetables
Sweets (candy, baked goods, etc.)	Fruit
Soda and juice	Blended smoothies made from whole fruits and vegetables
Frozen or fast-food chicken nuggets	Whole pieces of chicken or fish or fish sticks
Pasta and white rice	Brown rice, quinoa, farro, whole grain oat (oatmeal)

To make it easier to introduce new foods to picky eaters, you can use an approach called *food chaining*. With this approach, you use foods your child already likes to help them connect to new foods that are similar—making new links and lengthening the "chain." The key to making this approach successful is to understand the characteristics of the food that your child likes and consistently introduce new foods that are similar. For example, if they like banana because it's soft and sweet, you might try introducing ripe cantaloupe or peach, which have similar texture and sweetness. If your child likes Cheerios because they're small, round, and crunchy, you might try introducing edamame or nuts.

If your child is already eating a variety of nutrient-rich whole foods, it may be time to see whether eliminating certain foods is helpful. Elimination diets involve removing one or more food types from the diet at a time, and most diets touted for autism are elimination diets. There are also certain health conditions like life-threatening food allergies that make elimination necessary. But even without the diagnosis of a specific food allergy, there might be health benefits to removing certain foods from your child's diet. The gold standard approach to elimination diets is to methodically remove foods one at a time and record any changes in symptoms or behavior, and then to reintroduce them and note any changes in symptoms or behavior. This requires close tracking and is best done with the support of a medical professional who specializes in nutrition.

Adding nutrients to your child's diet by taking nutritional supplements could also help. This is most important when laboratory tests show that your child has a vitamin or mineral deficiency. Common nutrient deficiencies in autism include vitamin D and iron. Some research studies have also found lower levels of other vitamins and minerals in autism, including vitamin B12, vitamin B6, folate, and zinc. Depending on your child's medical history and diet, your doctor may recommend laboratory testing for these nutrients. Even if there's no deficiency on standard blood testing, nutritional supplements may be helpful for certain symptoms, as you learned in chapter 5.

Exploring dietary changes and supplementation in autism takes time and consistent effort. Partnering with a qualified medical professional can help your child get the most benefit.

EXERCISE

Exercise not only improves physical health, but it's also one of the best ways to support neurodevelopment. Many parents are surprised to learn that for autistic children, physical exercise improves social abilities, communication, emotion regulation, executive function, behavior, coordination, physical strength, endurance, anxiety, sleep, gut health, and overall quality of life. Exercise creates positive changes by enhancing mitochondrial health, reducing inflammation, and counteracting the effects of chronic stress. Exercise also increases the activity of natural chemicals like endorphins and brain-derived neurotrophic factor (BDNF) protein, which improve mental health and brain development.

If you'd like to make exercise part of your child's routine but aren't sure how, start with an activity they already enjoy that's within their current level of motor skill and stamina. I've seen children start by walking or jogging just a short distance and work their way up to running a 5K race. I've seen children flourish in swimming, bicycling, rock climbing, hiking, paddleboarding, weight lifting, skiing, CrossFit, and many other athletic activities. Seeing others enjoy these activities—whether live or on videos—can encourage your child's interest. Set your child up for success by starting with short periods of participation and gradually increasing duration and intensity.

The benefits of exercise come with consistency, and having support from friends, family, instructors, or therapists makes a big difference. Few things in life inspire joy like recreation and sports. Since we know these types of activities can also improve social skills, communication, behavior, anxiety, depression, inattention, sleep disturbance, learning, memory, and so much more, I recommend making enjoyable exercise a top priority.

RELATIONSHIPS

Even though autism affects how someone interacts socially, it doesn't mean that autistic people don't want to connect with other people. In fact, the opposite is true. Autistic people desire human connection, but social interaction is a complex behavior that requires us to rapidly process sensory information while also coordinating cognitive, language, and motor functions—you'll learn why all these are needed for social interaction later in this chapter. Because of this, social interaction can easily cause overstimulation and anxiety, especially when groups of people are involved.

To help your child build positive, caring relationships without overstimulation and anxiety, start with the important people in their life. These could be family members, friends, teachers, therapists, coaches, or other caregivers. Observe if your child is comfortable in their presence. See if these people understand how to interact in ways that aren't overstimulating and if they bring a positive energy that helps your child feel confident and capable. Pay particular attention to any behaviors by others that seem to have a negative effect on your child.

Akian Chaifetz was ten years old and a student at New Jersey's Horace Mann Elementary School when school staff began telling his father that Akian was having violent outbursts. This was shocking to his father because Akian usually had a gentle manner, so he became concerned that things might be happening at school to upset Akian. He placed a recording device on Akian and found that he was being verbally and emotionally abused at school by a teacher and a teacher's aide. Akian was spoken to in degrading ways and exposed to inappropriate conversations about alcohol and sex. School staff called him a "bastard" and said to him, "Go ahead and scream because guess what? You're going to get nothing until your mouth is shut." This example is one that we know about because Akian's father took the extra step of getting to the root cause of his son's behavior change, but for every example that comes to light, there are likely so many more that remain hidden.

For children who are still early in the process of developing social skills, it's essential to remove negative interactions with people and replace them with positive ones. One-to-one or small-group interactions are less likely to overwhelm your child's sensory processing capabilities and more likely to offer opportunities for them to get to know others in a deeper way. Having a skilled therapist or instructor to facilitate interactions can also help.

STRESS

Stress affects both the body and mind. We experience stress when we perceive something as threatening. Threats activate the sympathetic branch of the autonomic nervous system and increase activity of stress hormones (like cortisol and adrenaline). The stress response—or "fight, flight, freeze" response—can also involve negative thoughts and emotions. In the short term, stress prepares you to respond quickly to urgent situations. But in the long term, stress has negative effects on just about every part of the body.

We know that elevated stress is common in autism. Difficulty with sensory processing can make stimuli from the environment feel unpredictable and threatening. Stress can also be triggered by repetitive thoughts, social interactions, demands to carry through with tasks that are beyond a child's current skill level, and difficulty communicating needs and preferences. We can take steps to help in each of these areas. Reducing sensory stimulation, modifying task demands, and providing communication support are all important. Providing information to address any worries your child may have and offering positive statements can reduce distressing, repetitive thoughts. General strategies like physical exercise, listening to music, spending time in nature, or engaging in arts and crafts, meditation, or prayer can all help. Living in today's world brings stress to all of us, and you've probably developed strategies for managing your own stress. What helps you may have the potential to help your child, so use your own experiences to guide you.

Our bodies also experience biological stress from exposure to industrial chemicals, pollutants, and other toxins in the environment. Research has shown that some of these chemicals can interfere with brain development and may be contributing to the increase in neurodevelopmental diagnoses, including autism, ADHD, and others. These chemicals are widespread in our environment, and reducing exposure is not always possible. When parents ask me what they can do, I encourage them to explore reputable sources for more information like the Environmental Working Group (ewg.org).

Building Brain Networks

Once the conditions in the body are in place for neurodevelopment, you can make progress in building brain networks in the six major developmental domains: sensory, motor, cognitive, language, social, and emotional. This begins by understanding your child's current abilities in each domain and then building new abilities with the just-right challenge. In this section we'll walk step-by-step through each domain, starting with your child's sensory profile.

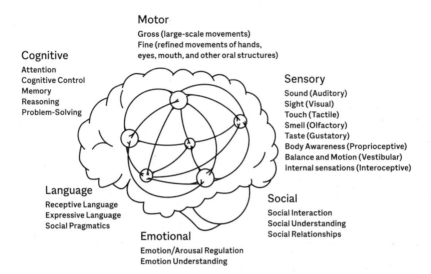

Motor
Gross (large-scale movements)
Fine (refined movements of hands,
eyes, mouth, and other oral structures)

Cognitive
Attention
Cognitive Control
Memory
Reasoning
Problem-Solving

Sensory
Sound (Auditory)
Sight (Visual)
Touch (Tactile)
Smell (Olfactory)
Taste (Gustatory)
Body Awareness (Proprioceptive)
Balance and Motion (Vestibular)
Internal sensations (Interoceptive)

Language
Receptive Language
Expressive Language
Social Pragmatics

Social
Social Interaction
Social Understanding
Social Relationships

Emotional
Emotion/Arousal Regulation
Emotion Understanding

SENSORY

The brain, one could argue, exists to perceive. After all, we couldn't experience the world without sensory perception. All living organisms sense their environment, but not in the same ways. The animal kingdom offers fascinating examples of different sensory abilities. Bats, for example, can hear ultrasonic sounds that humans can't. This helps them navigate their environment and hunt prey. Boa constrictors, pythons, and other snakes can detect thermal radiation (heat) emitted by the bodies of other animals. Bees can sense magnetic fields and use the earth's magnetic field to guide their movements. All living things experience the world in different ways based on their sensory systems.

A human's sensory system includes special sensors called *receptors* within the skin, eyes, ears, nose, and mouth, as well as a few others that you may not have heard of.

Special cells in the inner ear detect balance and movement
(*vestibular* sense).

Special neurons within muscle, tendons, and joints detect body position (*proprioceptive* sense).

Signals from organs in the body travel to the brain with messages about hunger, thirst, temperature, and pain (*interoceptive* sense).

When information from sensory receptors reaches the brain, it travels to different areas of the cortex for processing. Our senses are constantly sending information to the brain. The brain sorts through this information, determines what's important, and then decides how to respond.

Sensory differences are considered core features of autism. A child may show increased sensitivity to everyday sounds, like blenders, vacuum cleaners, or babies crying, or may have trouble tolerating certain lights, types of clothing, or food textures. This is referred to as *hypersensitivity or over-responsivity*. Autistic author and comedian Michael McCreary describes it this way in his book *Funny, You Don't Look Autistic*:

> *When I was first diagnosed with ASD [autism spectrum disorder], I didn't feel that different from other kids. But I did know one thing: my senses were heightened. . . . My socks and the tags in my clothes continued to drive me crazy. . . . Chewing sounded louder to me. Axe Body Spray smelled worse. And I could not do crowds. My dad took me to my first hockey game when I was six. I can't remember who was playing, but I'll never forget the crowd's cheers after the home team scored. I crumpled to the floor. . . . I couldn't help it. I was having a sensory overload, which is what happens when there's too much stimulation coming at you at once.*

Sensory differences can also include reduced responses to sensory input. This could be a reduced response to pain, a reduced awareness of how one's body is positioned or how it's moving, or a reduced sense of body temperature, hunger, or fullness. This is called *hyposensitivity or under-responsivity.* An autistic person may also show a unique interest in certain sensory aspects of the environment, such as smelling, touching, or looking at things in a particular way.

As more research is done and more autistic people share their experiences, we're learning that the sensory differences in autism seem to be driving many autistic behaviors. A child who rocks, twirls, jumps, runs, or climbs may be seeking information about body movement or body position. A child who looks at things from the corner of their eyes or turns on and off lights may be seeking visual stimulation. A child who insists on following a certain routine may do so because changing the routine brings unexpected sensory stimulation that's harder to process and more stressful. A person who avoids group social interactions and crowds may do so because the sensory information is overwhelming. Some research studies have found that sensory perception is already altered in young infants who years later are diagnosed with autism. Some infants may be quiet and less active because they are hyposensitive (so-called "easy" babies) and others may be more irritable because they are hypersensitive (so-called "difficult" babies).

Understanding Your Child's Sensory Profile

SOUND (AUDITORY)

Does your child show signs of being more sensitive to certain sounds?

Sounds in large gatherings, restaurants, gyms, or malls bother your child.

Sounds from blenders, vacuums, lawn mowers, or other machines bother your child.

Other sounds bother your child (e.g., dogs barking, babies crying, alarms, whistles, etc.).

Does your child show signs of being less sensitive to certain sounds?

Your child doesn't notice sounds that others notice.

Your child doesn't respond when their name is called.

Your child needs spoken instructions to be repeated and responds more consistently when spoken to in a loud voice.

Your child likes to raise the volume of music or television.

Does your child show signs of experiencing sound in unique ways?

Your child shows a strong interest in sounds that others don't notice.

Your child likes making repeated sounds, like humming or other vocalizations, or uses other objects to make repeated sounds, like flushing a toilet.

SIGHT (VISUAL)

Does your child show signs of being more sensitive to vision?

Your child is bothered by bright light or by certain types of lighting (e.g., strobe lights, flickering lights, or fluorescent lights).

Your child gets overwhelmed or distracted in places filled with colors, objects, or people to look at.

Your child seeks out areas that are darkened (with less light).

Does your child show signs of being less sensitive to vision?

Your child may not notice items around them that others notice.

Does your child show signs of experiencing their vision in unique ways?

Your child looks intently at things with a unique appearance, like reflective surfaces, interesting patterns, or moving objects or body parts.

TOUCH (TACTILE)

Does your child show signs of being more sensitive to touch?

Your child is bothered by being touched lightly or unexpectedly, by being touched on their face, by the feel of new clothes, by having their fingernails or toenails cut, or when crumbs are around their mouth.

Your child avoids touching messy things (like paint or glue), doesn't like having messy hands, or dislikes brushing their teeth.

Your child is bothered by fuzzy or furry textures or by different food textures (slimy food, food with a combination of textures, etc.).

Does your child show signs of being less sensitive to touch?

Your child isn't bothered by sensations others would find painful and doesn't cry when seriously hurt.

Your child has trouble finding things in a bag, backpack, or drawer without looking or needs to look at their hands when using them for a task.

Your child doesn't seem to notice when they're being touched or doesn't seem to feel contact with items, like saliva or food on their face or lips.

Does your child show signs of experiencing touch in unique ways?

Your child often explores objects by touching and feeling them.

Your child touches people, sometimes more than others would like.

Your child puts nonfood items in their mouth.

TASTE (GUSTATORY)

Does your child show signs of being more sensitive to taste?

Your child is bothered by the taste of many foods.

Your child avoids tasting unfamiliar foods or eats only certain brands of food.

Does your child show signs of being less sensitive to taste?

Your child doesn't show much of a preference between different foods or flavors.

Your child prefers foods with strong flavors (e.g., bitter, sour, or spicy).

SMELL (OLFACTORY)

Does your child show signs of being more sensitive to smell?

Your child notices scents or odors that others don't.

Your child is bothered by smells that don't bother others.

Your child gags or vomits at certain smells or avoids public restrooms because of the smell.

Does your child show signs of being less sensitive to smell?

Your child doesn't notice strong or unusual smells.

Your child isn't bothered by smells that bother others.

Does your child show signs of experiencing smell in unique ways?

Your child smells new objects or items before using them or smells objects when playing with them.

BODY AWARENESS (PROPRIOCEPTIVE)

Does your child show signs of reduced body awareness?

Your child holds objects like utensils or writing instruments too loosely or tightly to use easily.

Your child uses too much force or pressure for a task, like slamming doors or pushing too hard on objects, which may cause things to break.

Your child seeks activities that involve pushing, pulling, dragging, jumping, hanging off things, crashing, or rough play.

Your child often spills or knocks over items.

Your child bangs their head or other body parts or pushes their body against walls, objects, or people.

Your child takes excessive risks during play (like jumping off furniture, climbing very high, etc.).

BALANCE AND MOTION (VESTIBULAR)

Does your child show signs of being more sensitive to motion?

Your child avoids swings and slides.

Your child does not like to try new physical activities and prefers sedentary activities.

Does your child show signs of being less sensitive to motion?

Your child rocks, sways, or squirms when seated.

Your child prefers to be in motion, like spinning, swinging, or rolling.

Does your child show signs of experiencing motion and balance in unique ways?

Your child has trouble with balance and may avoid walking on uneven surfaces.

Your child avoids tilting their head backward.

Your child has difficulty coordinating both sides of the body.

Your child has trouble looking at something while their head is moving, like running and catching a ball at the same time.

Your child is bothered by being upside down or has a strong preference to be upside down.

INTERNAL SENSATIONS (INTEROCEPTIVE)

Does your child show signs of being more sensitive to internal body sensations?

Your child is much more irritable on days when they have more gas and/or haven't had a recent bowel movement.

Your child's mood and/or behavior decline significantly when they're hungry, thirsty, too hot, or too cold.

Does your child show signs of being less sensitive to internal body sensations?

Your child seems less aware of body sensations like hunger, thirst, heat, or cold.

Your child seems less aware of the need to use the toilet.

Your child doesn't seem bothered by hunger, thirst, heat, or cold.

MOTOR

Just as organisms perceive the world differently based on their sensory systems, they also move differently based on their motor systems. Consider the slowness of a turtle or the speed of a cheetah. Think about the way a hummingbird hovers or a snake slithers. Humans have found ways to hone the motor system to perform exquisite acts of musical performance, dance, athletics, and acrobatics.

The motor system is extraordinary, but it's not independent. It relies on sensory information to function. Have you ever had part of your body go numb, maybe from sitting in a position for too long or after getting numbing medicine for a dental procedure? It's harder to move a part of your body that you can't feel. When your mouth is numb, you have trouble talking. When your leg is numb, you have trouble walking. When the sensory information coming into the brain is absent, unreliable, or not processed appropriately in the brain, the motor system has trouble planning, coordinating, and carrying out movement.

On the flip side, what we sense from the environment is also determined by how we move. The brain receives very different sensory stimuli when you're jumping than when you're standing still, when your eyes are darting from place to place than when they're scanning slowly, and even when you're sucking on a gumball than when you're chewing it. That's why therapists, doctors, and psychologists often combine the words *sensory* and *motor* into a single term: *sensory-*

motor or *sensorimotor*. Our sensory and motor systems have separate roles, but they're completely integrated and interdependent.

Our motor system includes brain regions that plan movements (*association cortex*), brain regions that directly signal muscles how to move (*primary motor cortex*), and nerves that carry the information between the brain and muscles (*corticospinal tract* and *peripheral nerves*). In the motor system, some parts of the brain influence the pace, smoothness, and coordination of movement, while others influence how easy it is to start and stop movements or to switch between different movements.

Some movements are voluntary, meaning within a person's control, like kicking a ball, picking up a grocery bag, or typing on a keyboard. Other movements are involuntary, like the movements that occur during seizures, the small trembling movements of the hands that some people get as they age, and the jerks of the body that happen during sleep. Most of the movement differences in autism are considered semi-voluntary. These are movements that a person can control to some degree but not completely. The word *stereotypy* is used for repeated movements that follow a fixed, stereotyped pattern. When a behavior repeats itself, we know it's because the underlying brain network is firing in a repeated way. Sometimes professionals use the informal term "stuck loop" for a brain network that's causing a repetitive behavior. We know that these can happen outside of a person's awareness, as though on autopilot. Just as some people bounce their leg, twirl their hair, or fidget in other ways without noticing it, autistic people may not notice their repetitive behaviors. Controlling these behaviors may divert attention and energy away from other activities, and some autistic people have said that repetitive behaviors have a calming effect and that stopping them can lead to increased anxiety.

Another motor difference in autism is difficulty planning and executing sequences of movements, which is called *dyspraxia* or *apraxia* (these terms are interchangeable). In essence, behaviors are sequences of movements, and repetitive behaviors and apraxia are, in some ways, two sides of the same coin. Because apraxia makes learning new movement sequences more difficult, there's a tendency to repeat the same familiar sequences. And when someone's behavioral repertoire is limited to the same repeated sequences, there are fewer opportunities to practice and develop other motor sequences.

A promising research area looking at the motor system in autism uses eye-tracking technology to measure children's eye movements. These sophisticated measurements of a child's eye movements can aid early autism diagnosis and help track a child's developmental progress over time. Advances in eye-tracking technology are especially exciting because they offer a way to objectively measure motor system activity and to use this data to supplement subjective developmental assessments, which rely on caregivers' and professionals' observations of children's behavior.

Understanding Your Child's Motor Profile

What are your child's gross motor skills (large body movements)?

Roll from back to belly and belly to back

Sitting

Crawling

Walking

Running

Going up and down stairs

Kicking a ball

Jumping

Hopping

Throwing

Catching

Skipping

Hiking

Jump rope

Riding a bike

Climbing on playground equipment

Swimming, rock climbing, or other athletic activities

What can your child do with their hands (fine motor skills)?

Clapping

Picking up small items and holding them between the thumb
    and one finger

Stacking blocks or other toys

Turning pages

Holding a crayon, pen, or pencil and using it to scribble, draw, or
    write

Finger painting

Removing food from a wrapper

Turning a doorknob

Opening and closing containers

Putting on or taking off shoes

Using scissors

Painting with a brush

Getting dressed and undressed

Making shapes out of playdough

Turning on and off a faucet

Washing hands

Brushing teeth

Cutting and gluing materials for arts and crafts

Tying shoelaces

Sewing

Playing a musical instrument

Helping around the house (e.g., washing dishes, folding laundry, cleaning, cooking, etc.)

What sounds can your child make?

Vowel sounds (e.g., *a, e, i, o, u*)
Consonant sounds (e.g., *g, t, p, m, l, k,* etc.)
One-syllable sounds or words (e.g., *ma, da, no*)
Multisyllable sounds and words
Two-word or three-word phrases
Sentences

What can your child eat and swallow?

Liquids
Yogurt
Pureed foods (like applesauce)
Soft foods like oranges, berries, peaches, rice, and pasta
Crunchy foods like crackers, chips, nuts, apples, and raw vegetables
Meat
Multiple textures in a single bite

How does your child use their eyes?

To track objects
To get around the house, school, and other settings
To look for things they need
To watch videos
To read
To make art
To play sports

COGNITIVE

Cognition is about how we think. It includes a broad set of skills, like attention, memory, comprehension, reasoning, problem-solving, and imagination. Unlike the sensory and motor systems, which have nerves in the brain and throughout the rest of the body, the entire cognitive system is in the brain. The frontal lobes play a particularly important role in cognitive processes, and connections between the frontal lobes and other parts of the brain allow our thoughts to influence our senses, our movements, and all other brain functions.

Some of the most important findings to emerge from autism research involve cognitive differences. The core autistic feature of behavioral inflexibility comes from differences in *cognitive control*. Cognitive control refers to the mental ability driven by the prefrontal cortex that enables a person to control their behavior rather than respond in automatic or impulsive ways. Cognitive control includes these components:

Initiating (starting a new action or thought)
Inhibiting (stopping an action or thought)
Sustaining (maintaining an action or thought)
Switching (transitioning between different actions or thoughts)

The prefrontal cortex gathers information about the current situation, considers what response to prioritize, and directs the activity of neural networks—like the conductor of an orchestra directs musicians on when and how to play.

Cognitive control directs our attention, and in doing so shapes how we perceive the world. The autistic brain tends to direct more attention to details than to the bigger picture—to parts rather than the whole. In cognitive neuroscience this is called enhanced *local processing* and reduced *global processing*. This cognitive style lends itself to retaining large amounts of data and has its benefits, including an astonishing ability to recall facts from both recent and distant memory (also called *short-term* and *long-term memory*). But it may come at the expense of seeing how pieces come together to create a bigger picture.

To teach this concept to doctors and therapists at Cortica, I show them these images used in neuropsychological assessments of local and global processing:

They tell me in the first image, they see a heart made of stars, and in the second, the letter *M* made of *T*s. I explain that in this simple task, they've used both their local processing skills to discern the parts (the stars and the *T*s) and global processing skills to see the whole (the heart and the *M*).

Then I show them the photo of a person's face and ask, "If you had enhanced local processing and reduced global processing, what would you see?"

"The parts of the face," they say. The ears, lips, eyebrows—but not the whole face all together.

"Would that make it harder to recognize faces and harder to identify emotions from facial expressions?" I ask.

"Yes," they say, nodding. They're beginning to see autism in a new way.

Difficulty with facial recognition—or what neurologists call *prosopagnosia*—affects about one-third of autistic people, compared to 1 to 2 percent of non-autistic people. People with prosopagnosia often have difficulty recognizing even close friends and family members. They develop coping strategies, like learning to recognize people based on a particular facial feature or the sound of their voice. They sometimes cope by avoiding people. Simple steps could make a big difference—like wearing a name badge or saying your name each time you meet (as you might when calling someone on the phone).

To help new doctors and therapists at Cortica deepen their understanding of cognitive control and get a sense of what it feels like to engage their cognitive control skills in a challenging task, I present them with another task used in cognitive assessments called the Stroop task. I have them look at a list of words, "red, green, yellow, red, yellow, green, red," and so on. The words name different colors *and* the words themselves are also colored. So "green," for example, is written in yellow, red, or green. Sometimes the color of the word matches the word itself, and sometimes it doesn't. I give them the instruction to name the *color* not the word, and to do this as fast as they can.

Here's a version of the Stroop task for you to try using the colors black, gray, and white. Your job is to go from left to right, top to bottom, just as though you were reading, but instead of saying the word, name the color, and do this as fast as you can. (Name the color of the inside of the letters, not the outline.)

Black	White	Gray	Black	**White**
White	**Gray**	Black	**Black**	Gray
Gray	White	Black	White	**White**
Black	Gray	**White**	Gray	Black
White	**Black**	Gray	White	**White**

Here the word is a distraction. It makes it harder to pay attention to the color. To do this task you have to inhibit your brain's impulse to read the word and direct it to name the color. The Stroop task is designed to challenge your cognitive control skills. The task is set up to make it harder for your brain to do what's been asked. People feel slow, frustrated, and uncomfortable, and they make frequent errors. Some give up before they finish.

The reason I ask Cortica's doctors and therapists to do this task is so they can experience what one of their autistic clients might experience when asked to do a task that isn't designed for the way their brain works. The child may understand the instructions, have the knowledge required (like for this task, recognizing colors), and may want to do what you've asked. But something about the way the task is set up makes it hard for them to show their true abilities. That's why modifying tasks, offering supports, and trying new strategies based on an understanding of your child's neurodevelopmental profile is so important.

Cognition encompasses a vast array of mental abilities, including all your child's thoughts and memories. None of us can fully know what occupies another person's thoughts. But it's incredibly important not to assume the *absence* of thoughts, which is a mistake that's often made, especially for autistic people who have limited speech. Fortunately, many autistic people have been able to describe, years later, the thoughts, perceptions, and knowledge they had back when they couldn't yet speak.

One story that I'll never forget is from the dad of a ten-year-old nonspeaking girl who was just learning to communicate through typing. Her speed of typing was slow at first, and she made many errors, but her dad was thrilled by his daughter's progress and eagerly awaited every word and sentence that she produced. One morning, she started the day by typing to her dad, "Your breath stinks." This made her dad burst out in laughter (and pop a mint). Nothing felt better than getting a glimpse into his daughter's thoughts, no matter what the thoughts were.

The belief that a person most likely perceives and understands what's happening around them, even if they can't express it, is sometimes referred to as "assuming competence." This is one of the most important concepts for anyone who interacts with neurodivergent people to embrace. It means seeing others as capable and competent, with the capacity to learn and develop new abilities. At Cortica we use the phrase "recognizing competence" because there's now so much evidence showing competence and capability in autistic people, we don't have to assume it's there. We just need to recognize it.

Understanding Your Child's Cognitive Profile

What does your child pay attention to?

What helps your child pay attention?

What does your child seem to remember well?

What are some things you've seen your child figure out how to do?

What are some ways you've seen your child use their imagination?

What are some ideas your child has shared with you?

What are some things you've explained to your child that you can tell they've understood?

What are some topics your child has shown an interest in learning about?

What subjects has your child learned about—either with or without a teacher?

LANGUAGE

Language skills fall within two main categories: *receptive language* (the ability to understand language) and *expressive language* (the ability to use language to communicate). Although language is considered its own developmental domain, it relies almost entirely on sensory, motor, and cognitive skills. We receive language through our senses: we hear words that are spoken; we see words that are written or gestures used in sign language; and people who use the language system called braille feel the patterns of raised dots on a page through the sense of touch. To produce language, we use oral motor skills for speech production, the fine motor skills of the hands for writing and typing, and the gestures of sign language for signing. Both receptive and expressive language rely on cognitive functions. To understand what others are saying or what you're reading, for example, you need to pay attention to words and recall the meaning of those words from memory.

In the brain, specialized areas of the frontal lobe (called *Broca's area*) participate in expressive language, while areas of the temporal and parietal lobes (called *Wernicke's area*) engage in receptive language. This separation of roles means that someone who can't speak may be able to understand language. On the flip side, someone may be able to speak but not understand what other people are saying. This can be hard to imagine until you've seen it happen. Neurologists who treat stroke patients see this routinely. A stroke that injures Broca's area causes halting or absent speech but preserves the ability to understand speech (called *Broca's aphasia*). In contrast, following a stroke that injures Wernicke's area, a person may be able to speak with fluidity but not understand what they themselves or others are saying (called *Wernicke's aphasia*). These patterns are striking and surprising, until you know the neurology behind them.

Autistic author and comedian Michael McCreary describes how he often quoted lines from movies when he first started speaking at age three. He says, "I didn't necessarily know what I was saying; I just liked the way it sounded." But we also know that autistic children sometimes repeat scripts from movies to express something relevant to their present situation. Given these possibilities, it's important to allow your child to use language in this way. If you think the scripting is a sign of anxiety, which it sometimes is, try to address the anxiety. If you think it's a way of communicating, then see it as an opportunity to engage your child. Offer a response based on what you think your child means but also look for cues from your child to see how your responses are received. This can be a way to deepen your relationship and nurture your child's development, as it was for father and son Ron and Owen Suskind. As Ron describes in his book *Life, Animated*, Owen's passion for Disney movies led him to repeat scripts from these movies, which opened the door to communication with others.

About 30 percent of autistic children speak fewer than thirty words and are classified as "nonverbal." This label often leads to the mistaken assumption that a child does not understand language when, in fact, many do. Published autistic authors and many autistic children in my care have articulately described what others said to them when they didn't yet have a way to express themselves. Some of these people developed speech later, while others communicate mainly through written language. Replacing the term *nonverbal* with *nonspeaking* reminds us that someone who doesn't speak may very well understand what we're saying. Providing appropriate instruction to expand a child's receptive language is one of the best ways to support overall neurodevelopment, including the growth of expressive language.

Reading and writing are language abilities that rely on different brain networks than speaking does. When we hear others speak, the sounds are processed in brain regions near the ears called *auditory cortex*. But when we read, the visual images are processed in brain areas near the back of the head called *visual cortex*. For autistic people, processing sound (called *auditory processing*) is often more difficult than processing visual images (called *visual processing*). Research studies that track sound signals from the ears through the brain show that the signals travel more slowly and generate different patterns of brain activation in autistic people than they do in nonautistic people. Some autistic people have a hard time discerning speech sounds. For example, Temple Grandin describes being unable to hear consonants and able to hear only vowels in others' speech as a young child. In contrast, the ability to process and remember visual information is often enhanced in autism, leading some to have a photographic memory. This is why hyperlexia—the precocious ability to read words before age five without being taught—happens in as many as 20 percent of autistic children. Some researchers consider hyperlexia to be an early sign of autism since the vast majority of children with hyperlexia—84 percent, according to one study—meet diagnostic criteria for autism. Because many autistic children recognize words easily, pictures may not be necessary when using alternative communication approaches, even for children under age five. A picture shows only one example of what a word could mean, and pictures often can't accurately capture the meaning of action words (verbs), like *run* and *jump*, and other words with complex meanings.

There are also other reasons the autistic brain may be more suited to written language. Written words are stable—they remain on the page or screen and aren't fleeting like speech sounds. Sounds come and go quickly; if you aren't paying close attention, the words are gone. Speaking also presents greater motor challenges, requiring rapid, coordinated fine motor movements of the mouth, lips, tongue, and palate. In contrast, written language can be produced with simpler movements, like pointing to letters and words on a page or a screen or pushing keys on a keyboard.

We use language both in literal and nonliteral ways. For example, saying "I could eat a horse" is a nonliteral or indirect way of telling someone you're hungry, and saying "It's time to hit the sack" is a way of saying "Go to bed." People constantly use language in nonliteral ways, and this can be hard for autistic people to interpret. An unfortunate trend I've seen recently is for a parent to respond to a child's inappropriate behavior by saying "No, thank you," when they really mean "I don't want you to do that." Words or statements with multiple possible meanings also present challenges, especially when the intended meaning is implied rather than explicit. Sarcasm, for example, conveys meaning through context and tone of voice. In conversation, these nuances can be hard to follow. Helpful steps include speaking in clear, direct ways and finding ways to make the implicit explicit. If the other person doesn't understand what you've said, say it a different way. And consider whether writing it down might be even better.

Understanding Your Child's Language Profile

RECEPTIVE LANGUAGE

What are your child's skills for receiving and understanding language?

Auditory

What are examples of things you or others say (whether instructions, statements, or questions) that your child understands?

Visual

What are examples of things your child reads and understands?

What are examples of signs or gestures your child understands?

What visual images (e.g., pictures or videos) does your child understand?

EXPRESSIVE LANGUAGE

What are your child's skills for producing language?

Oral Motor Skills

What is your child able to say that's easily understood by others?

Are there ways your child adjusts their speech volume, intonation, and pace to help them express what they mean?

Fine Motor Skills (e.g., fingers, hands, wrists)

What can your child express through handwriting?

What can your child express by pointing to letters on a letterboard to spell words?

What can your child express by typing (with one or more fingers)?

What can your child express by pointing to or selecting words or pictures?

SOCIAL PRAGMATICS
(USE OF LANGUAGE FOR SOCIAL INTERACTION)

Are there ways your child adjusts their communication based on the social context (e.g., who is present, the relationship they have with those present, relevant past events, the current setting, or other social factors)?

SOCIAL

Social development includes a broad set of skills that help us interact with other people. Of all the domains of brain development, social development is the most misunderstood.

First, parents and professionals alike tend not to recognize that social development relies on underlying sensory, motor, cognitive, and language skills.

Social interaction relies on sensory perception. We need our senses to perceive what another person is saying or doing. Imagine trying to interact with another person if you couldn't see, hear, or touch them.

Social interaction relies on the motor system. Any interaction with another person requires movement of some part of the body, like the mouth, eyes, hands, or other body parts. Imagine trying to communicate something to another person without moving any part of your body.

Social interaction relies on cognitive skills. To interact socially we need to understand the context of the interaction and what can and should take place.

Social interaction usually involves language. This may be in the form of speech, writing, or gestures.

When parents tell me they'd like help improving their child's social skills, what they're asking for, but often don't realize, is help building the sensory, motor, cognitive, and language skills that enable social interaction.

Another common misconception has to do with the reasons why autistic people engage in fewer social interactions. People tend to think this has to do with a lack of desire for relationships or social connection, but that isn't the case. More often it's because social interactions are complex. They require the coordination of many sensory, motor, cognitive, and language skills. Autistic people have also described being unsure how to respond in social situations because they see many possible meanings and potential outcomes to a social interaction. Autistic people might also choose to spend time alone because of a history of maltreatment from others. Recognizing that these are all possibilities is important as you take actions to support your child's social development.

Neuroscientists sometimes use the term "social brain" to refer to areas of the brain that are important for social interaction. The social brain has been called a "complex super-network" because it involves so many regions and networks within the brain. The fact that social development is a composite of so many other abilities has raised questions about whether autism should be defined by social criteria. Many brain conditions affect social interaction in some way—like stroke,

Parkinson's, Alzheimer's, and Huntington's disease—but we don't define them by social or behavioral criteria. We define them by how they affect movement or cognition or by a specific biological cause or mechanism. The same should be the goal for defining autism. Doing so could advance our understanding of autism subtypes, which could transform how we approach autism research and therapies.

Understanding Your Child's Social Profile

What are examples of how your child initiates interactions with other people? Does your child approach others, look at them, speak to them, make physical contact, etc.?

How does your child respond when another person initiates an interaction? Does your child look at them, move closer to them, speak to them, make physical contact, etc.?

Who does your child interact with (e.g., family, friends, strangers, adults, older children, same-age peers, younger children)?

Does your child play interactively with other children?

Does your child take turns in conversations?

Are there ways your child uses facial expressions during interactions with others?

Does your child show or give items to others?

How does your child show concern for others?

How does your child show their sense of humor?

What are the important social relationships in your child's life?

EMOTIONAL

Emotional development is closely linked to social development, and the two are often referred to as one: *social-emotional development*. Neuroscientists think of emotions as subjective experiences that have a mental and physical component. They involve thoughts along with physiological changes in the body. Often these experiences generate behavioral responses, like outward expressions of joy, sadness, or anger.

A broad set of brain networks activate when we experience emotions. But one small structure called the *amygdala* has a notable role. The amygdala is a tiny structure in the brain, about the size of a pea, that evaluates sensory information from the surroundings and coordinates emotional responses. Brain networks that connect to the amygdala are among the many networks that function in unique ways in autism.

Subjective emotional experiences are hard to study, especially in people who have difficulty with expressive language. Research studies have found that some autistic people have difficulty identifying emotions in themselves and others (alexithymia), while others do not. The biggest takeaway is that we shouldn't make assumptions about the emotional experiences of others. This means we should not label others' emotions based on what we observe in their behavior. For example, a child who is throwing objects or hitting may not be feeling angry. A child who is crying may not be feeling sad. In the book *Sincerely, Your Autistic Child*, Dusya Lyubovskaya describes a tendency she had as a child to cry when she saw babies:

> When I was six years old and taking a walk with my mother, a
> woman who lived on the next block approached us and showed us
> her newborn, and I started crying and this woman thought that I

was jealous, and I was not able to communicate that I just did not find babies that exciting.

She also says,

I did not like and was irritated when adults made assumptions about why they thought I was crying. Instead of asking what was wrong or if I wanted a glass of water or any other thing that I could have had, they instead made assumptions, guessed, or had already made up their minds about why I was crying.

Having your emotions mislabeled by others can cause frustration and reduce trust in relationships.

Even if you're not sure what emotions your child is experiencing, you can still respond in a supportive way. Start by making a neutral statement that describes what just happened. For example, "We're on a walk, and now there's a baby here with us. I see you're crying." Then express your desire to understand what your child is experiencing: "I want to know how you're feeling. You can tell me if you like." Then pause to give your child time to respond. Offer your child support for communication. For example, if your child doesn't speak, you can offer their communication device or write a few words on a piece of paper, like "sad," "uncomfortable," "scared," "good," or "something else." You can say, "You might be feeling . . ." and then point to each of the words as you say them. Allow your child to look at the words and then wait to see if they point to one. Whichever option they select, or even if they don't select one, you can follow this up by offering them a choice about what to do next. For example, "We can leave, or we can stay." Or you can provide more options, like having a drink of water, eating a snack, going to another location, or having some time alone in a comfortable space. The key is to give your child a chance to express their emotions, while offering support for their communication, and then give them a choice for how they'd like to move on.

Building your child's skills for recognizing emotions and managing how they respond to emotions can be done through a number of approaches. The most effective techniques use a cognitive element in which you or another adult help develop your child's understanding of body sensations, thoughts, and behavioral responses associated with emotions. This should include opportunities for your child to use the words and concepts that they associate with emotions, which may be different from neurotypical constructs. Effective approaches also teach strategies for regulating stress that can accompany certain emotions.

Understanding Your Child's Emotional Profile

What are some ways your child expresses emotions (through words, movements, facial expressions, etc.)?

How does your child respond when you or others show different emotions (happiness, sadness, anger, etc.)?

In what situations is your child more likely to be calm, relaxed, and emotionally well-regulated?

In what situations is your child likely to show emotional dysregulation, and what does this look like?

Building Brain Networks
with the Just-Right Challenge

With your understanding of your child's profile in the six domains of neurodevelopment, you're ready to support their growth in each domain. You can do this by creating the just-right challenge in everyday activities and finding supportive therapists and other professionals to partner with you.

As you learned in chapter 4, the just-right challenge is a task slightly above your child's current skill level. With support, your child can carry out the task, and with additional practice, your child can do the task by themselves. This individualized challenge creates an optimal situation for learning and allows your child to go just beyond their current performance level without feeling frustrated.

THE NOT-RIGHT CHALLENGE

To start, let's consider some examples of non-optimal learning situations.

A task or activity that your child can already do independently without support falls into this category. That doesn't mean they should stop doing the activity; it just means the activity should no longer be treated as the focus of instruction. For example, if your child is independently brushing their teeth, getting dressed, and using the bathroom, they should continue to do all these things in their daily routines. Don't do things for your child that they can do for themselves. Instead, give your child plenty of opportunities to practice their skills so that they become more fluid and efficient and so the brain networks for those skills continue to be strengthened. But to advance neurodevelopment, your child will need new challenges.

Another not-right challenge is a task or activity that your child cannot do, even with support. This kind of demand can lead anyone to feel frustrated and experience a sense of failure, and this is especially true for autistic children who constantly face environments set up for neurotypical minds. In these scenarios you're likely to end up completing the task for your child, which can make them feel incapable. You may not know in advance if an activity falls within this category, but if you attempt it and see your child become frustrated, avoidant, or passive, adjust the task so that it's closer to your child's current skill level.

There may be activities that your child can do with support but, because of biological factors, isn't likely to progress in. For example, a child with permanent hearing loss should not be working on skills that train hearing. Instead, they should be working on other ways to receive information. This is tricky when the biological factors are less clear, which is often the case in autism. For example, we may not know if a child's neurobiology will allow for speech development. When this is the case, it's important to provide learning opportunities to promote speech while also teaching other means of communication that may be more accessible, like reading, writing, and using an assistive communication device. If your child has received appropriate treatment for co-occurring medical conditions and appropriate instruction and they're not advancing in a particular area of development, it's important to explore different ways to help them progress.

START WITH WHAT YOU KNOW

Parents sometimes tell me they're frustrated by what they don't understand about their child. I assure you that what you know far exceeds what you don't know. But it can be hard to appreciate what you know when you have a long list of unanswered questions. I ask the parents I work with to let go of the "I don't know" mentality, and this is what I hope you'll do, too. You've already begun the process by doing the exercises in this chapter to understand your child's developmental profile. These exercises are based on your observations and your knowledge about your child, and they should help you appreciate how much you already know. If your child has had professional evaluations by doctors, psychologists, or therapists to assess their development, this information can supplement your own. The developmental profile you've created for your child focuses on your observations and your knowledge of your child's strengths and abilities. Professionals offer an important perspective, too, but their view of your child's development should not overshadow yours.

LOOK AT EVERYDAY ACTIVITIES
THROUGH A DEVELOPMENTAL LENS

For your child to succeed in just about any activity, they'll need to use brain networks across all developmental domains. Skilled therapists with an understanding of neurodevelopment can quickly determine the sensory, motor, cognitive, language, social, and emotional demands of any activity. They can then adjust the activity so that the challenges within a particular domain—and combined across all domains—are within a child's reach. This is also something you can learn to do for your child, like the parents you'll see in these examples did for theirs.

Michelle, mom of Leon,
a three-year-old boy learning to follow two-step directions
Leon says about twenty words, but he doesn't say any phrases or sentences. His mom, Michelle, feels he understands a lot more than

he can say. Leon follows many familiar one-step directions, like "Give me the cup," "Bring me your shoes," "Put the toy here," and "Open your lunch box." Now Michelle thinks he may be ready to learn to follow two-step directions, and she wants to give it a try.

Here are relevant parts of Leon's neurodevelopmental profile:

Sensory

Auditory: Leon has reduced sensitivity to others' speech. He doesn't respond to his name being called or follow directions unless the person is close to him and speaks to him in a confident, clear voice.

Tactile: Leon has reduced sensitivity to touch. He doesn't seem to notice if someone is touching him unless the touch is firm and paired with seeing or hearing the person.

Motor

Fine motor: Leon can use his hands in many ways. He can pick up small items like coins; he can open containers, like a box of raisins or a plastic sandwich box; and he can use a crayon to draw on a piece of paper.

Cognitive

Attention: Leon can pay attention during one-to-one activities with a therapist or parent for up to five minutes at a time.

Working memory: Leon can remember and imitate two-step movements that he has seen others do, like clapping his hands and then spinning around.

Language

Receptive: Leon follows many familiar one-step directions.

Social

Leon spends more time with his mother than his father and
tends to follow directions more consistently from his mother.

Emotional

Regulation: Leon is usually calm and happy after he wakes up
from his afternoon nap. He often takes an afternoon walk
around the park near his home. Leon's emotional regulation
is best when he's outdoors and moving around.

Following a two-step direction is a challenge to Leon's cognitive
and receptive language abilities. He'll need to keep the information
he hears in his working memory and then follow the directions in
sequence, which is something he's never done before. To support his
success in this new challenge, Michelle keeps the other aspects of the
task—sensory, motor, social, and emotional—as simple as possible.
She picks a weekday afternoon to start, and she knows Leon's energy
and attention will be best during their afternoon walk around the
park. She prepares by writing down the two-step directions she wants
to teach Leon that day and puts the items she'll need into a bag. She
chooses the following two-step directions because she knows that
Leon can carry out each part when given as a one-step direction.

Open the box and give me a raisin.
Get the bottle and put it on the table.
Put the bottle in the bag and then give me the bag.

Now she'll combine them, so he needs to remember both and
then carry them out in sequence.

When they get to the park, Michelle and Leon sit side by side at a
picnic table where they often sit for a break. She puts the box of rai-

sins on the table and then rests her hand firmly on Leon's shoulder and in a loud, clear voice says, "Leon, open the box and give me a raisin." Leon looks at her but does not reach for the box. She waits, knowing that Leon may need time to process the two-part instruction. Leon then reaches for the box and gives it to her. Michelle recognizes that Leon is trying to do what she asked but that he needs more support. The challenge she presented was a little too much, but she believes he can get there. She reduces the challenge by giving him a command she knows he can do. She gives Leon the box and says, "Open the box." He promptly opens the box. "Good," she says. Then she puts a raisin on a napkin on the table and says, "Give me the raisin." Leon promptly gives her the raisin. "Nice job," she says. Leon gets up and runs to the swings. Michelle pushes him on the swing for a few minutes, and then they walk back to the picnic table together.

Michelle says, "We're going to eat the raisins together now." She pauses, puts her hand on Leon's arm, waits until he looks at her, and then says slowly and clearly, "Open the box and give me a raisin." And Leon follows through just as she's asked! The two of them enjoy eating the box of raisins together. After eating the raisins, Leon runs to the swings. Michelle decides not to ask Leon to do the other two-step directions she'd planned, since he's done so well and clearly wants to play. Instead, she saves them for the next day. And she continues to look for more opportunities for Leon to expand his receptive language by practicing two-step directions and adding new words and new actions, in new settings, eventually with Leon's father and others giving the directions.

Liz, mom of Tara, a six-year-old girl learning to dress herself

Liz wants to teach her daughter Tara how to dress herself. The current routine involves Tara standing next to her bed while her mom puts her shirt, pants, and socks on for her. Tara moves her arms and legs to help, but she's never put on a shirt, pants, or socks by herself.

Here are relevant parts of Tara's neurodevelopmental profile:

Sensory

Tactile: Tara has tactile sensitivity. She prefers soft, loose cotton clothes, stretchy waistbands, and ankle socks. Seams and tags bother her. She's willing to wear more restrictive clothes, but only for short periods of time.

Visual: Tara likes to use her vision to examine objects. She often looks at the parts of toys or at interesting patterns on fabric.

Body awareness (proprioceptive): Tara has reduced body awareness. She likes crashing into things and playing rough. She often pushes her body against walls or lies on the ground.

Motor

Gross and fine motor: Tara can open and close drawers and pull clothes out from a drawer.

Cognitive

Attention: Tara can pay attention to activities with therapists and teachers for up to ten minutes at a time.

Language

Receptive: Tara follows many familiar one-step directions and some familiar two-step directions.

Emotional

Regulation: Tara usually wakes up well rested and well

regulated. But in the evening before bedtime, she's often tired, and that's when meltdowns are most likely.

With this information, Liz picks a morning to start. The night before, she sets up a small, sturdy chair in front of the full-length wall mirror in Tara's bedroom and makes sure several of Tara's favorite clothes are clean and folded in a drawer. In the morning she tells Tara to pick out a shirt and pants from the drawer. She stays close, ready to offer help, but sees that Tara doesn't need it. She then tells Tara to sit in the chair facing the mirror. Liz holds up the shirt so Tara can see it and says, "Today I want you to put this on by yourself. I can help if you need it, but I want you to try on your own." Liz says, "First, put your head in here," and points to the opening of the shirt. "Then put one arm in here," she says, pointing to the sleeve. "And then one arm in here," she says pointing to the other sleeve. She places the shirt flat on Tara's lap oriented with the front side down and the bottom opening near Tara's waist. Liz is ready to help move Tara's arms or hands if needed, but she knows to give the least amount of help that will still allow Tara to succeed. Liz needs to make only a few small adjustments to the position of the shirt, and Tara is able to do the rest by herself. Liz then proceeds with putting Tara's pants on for her, knowing that in a few days, once Tara is confident putting on her own shirt, they can begin working on pants, and then socks.

Since dressing posed a new motor challenge for Tara, Liz kept the language, cognitive, and sensory demands well within Tara's current level of skill. Liz supported Tara's body awareness by having her sit in a stable, sturdy chair. She also found ways for Tara's visual strength to support her success in learning this new skill by allowing her to look in a mirror and by drawing her attention to visual features of the clothes.

**Mark and Sheena, parents of John,
a thirteen-year-old boy learning to build friendships**

John's family moved to a new city, and he started seventh grade at a large public school where he didn't know anyone. A few months into the school year, his parents, Mark and Sheena, noticed that he hadn't made friends. John told his parents he ate lunch by himself. He also told his parents he was having a lot of "bad thoughts" and these thoughts made him feel sad and tired. When his parents asked him about the bad thoughts, he said they were about all the bad things that could happen, like forgetting to turn in his homework, getting a bad grade, saying something and having others laugh at him, or something bad happening to his parents.

Here are relevant parts of John's neurodevelopmental profile:

Sensory

Auditory and Visual: John feels a lot of stress when he's in
    crowds. He doesn't mind loud noises or seeing a lot of
    people around him, but when the two are combined he feels
    anxious and wants to leave the setting as quickly as possible.
    At his elementary school, John's teacher would set up a
    cardboard divider around his desk to help reduce visual
    stimuli. He was also allowed to wear sunglasses, earplugs,
    or headphones in class, which all helped him focus and
    self-regulate. Because he was doing so well after sixth grade,
    his parents didn't think he needed these strategies anymore,
    and he hasn't been using them.

Motor

Fine motor: John has exquisite fine motor skills when it comes
    to building intricate model cars, planes, or other vehicles.

He plays the piano and performs at recitals two or three times a year.

Cognitive

Attention: John can focus for several hours at a time if he's engaged in building something he likes.

Academic skills: He keeps up with the requirements of his general education seventh-grade class and doesn't receive any accommodations at his new school.

Language

Social pragmatics: John has difficulty with social pragmatics. He often misses sarcasm and has trouble figuring out if someone is joking with him or being serious. He tends to talk about his favorite topics and forgets to pause or ask people questions unless he's reminded to.

Social

John enjoys one-to-one time with other children his age or younger. He feels uncomfortable in groups and has a hard time following the rapid pace of conversation in a group of other children his age.

Emotional

John is happiest when he's building model vehicles.

He says that being depressed, sad, and tired all happen at the same time for him, and all these words describe how he's been feeling for the past few months.

Mark and Sheena realize that the current school setting is presenting too many challenges to John at once. The sensory challenges of being exposed to big, noisy crowds of students throughout the day is causing John increased stress. Even though he's keeping up with the cognitive requirements of his schoolwork, he's having to do this without accommodations for his auditory and visual sensitivities, which means the overall challenge he's facing is greater. Without one-to-one opportunities for socialization, he's missing out on social connection. The combined effect of all this is what John describes as being sad, tired, and depressed. His parents have noticed that he's so drained after school that he hasn't been able to practice the piano, and he's even been showing less interest in building model cars.

To reduce the overall challenge from John's school experience, his parents begin the process of setting up an individualized education program (chapter 9 includes more information on this). They plan to request the same accommodations that have helped John in the past. They also begin looking into other school options for him, recognizing that the social challenge at a large public school might be too much.

His parents also ask his piano teacher if she can match him with other students to play duets. They tell her that John tends to get along better with children a year or two younger than him. This gives John a chance to spend one-to-one time with other children with a shared interest. They also find an afterschool program that's centered on building projects using model kits. They enroll John in the program and tell the teachers in advance that they hope it can be an opportunity for John to get to know other children and develop friendships. The teachers decide they can encourage this by scheduling break times when John and one other child can spend time together, with one of the teachers nearby to help guide the interaction if needed. With the challenges at school reduced, and with new social opportunities that are set up to allow John to experience success, he feels happy and energized again.

FINDING SKILLED PARTNERS

When looking for professionals to support your child's development, the most important thing to know is that they can come from a variety of backgrounds. I've seen parents find great partners who have been trained in just about any discipline, some with decades of experience in autism services and many who were just starting out. What they have in common is the desire and ability to recognize competence in your child and the openness to learn about your child's unique neurodevelopmental profile.

Here are some therapeutic approaches you may want to consider. When you talk with potential partners, share your understanding of your child's development and ask how they would approach supporting your child's growth in each area.

Occupational Therapy (OT)

The *occupation* in *occupational therapy* refers to the activities that occupy our time. For adults, this includes self-care skills, work, and leisure activities. For children, occupational therapy focuses largely on self-care skills and play, since play is an essential part of childhood and an important way for children to gain new abilities.

OT is a well-established field that's made many exciting advances in recent decades in understanding and supporting autistic children. Thanks to Dr. A. Jean Ayres, the occupational therapist who defined the concept of the just-right challenge, and to other pioneers in the field of sensory processing, today's occupational therapists generally have a strong understanding of the sensory and motor foundations of child development. This gives them a central role in therapy programs for most autistic children.

Many children receive OT support in school, and parents sometimes assume that because their child receives some level of OT in school, they don't need additional OT services, but this usually isn't the case. Schools are often limited in the amount and type of OT they can offer, and there's usually a focus on academic goals with little or no support for building sensory processing skills. For many autistic children, there's a role for school-based OT as well as OT services outside of school to target a wider range of goals.

Music Therapy

Many families haven't heard of music therapy for autism, or have heard of it but may not see it as a service their child needs. Many parents mistakenly think the purpose of music therapy is to teach children how to play musical instruments. Although playing instruments might be part of music therapy, this isn't the focus. The focus of music therapy is to help a child strengthen a wide range of sensory, motor, cognitive, language, social, and emotional skills that promote success in daily life. Music therapists use the tools of music, including instruments, songs, rhythm, and intonation, to support a child's development across all domains.

Not all music therapy is equal. Just as with any other therapy, music therapy has a variety of approaches. But music therapists with a strong knowledge base in neurodevelopment are uniquely capable of supporting autistic children in every domain of development. That's because music has the power to stimulate brain networks across all developmental domains. Autistic children often respond positively to music by becoming more attentive, engaged, and well regulated. Brain imaging studies that measure brain activity when listening to music show that music can stimulate many brain regions simultaneously—more so than just about any other type of stimulus. You've probably experienced the way music can instill the almost irresistible urge to move your body (a sign of motor network activation). Music stirs our emotions and facilitates social bonds with others. Music also engages our attention and memory. People some-times think music is entertainment and can't be a serious therapeutic approach, but research shows that music profoundly influences brain activity and brain structure. For these reasons, music therapy is one of the most powerful tools for fostering child brain development, es-pecially in autism. Unfortunately, it's also the therapy that I see par-ents most often misunderstand and deprioritize. But for those who make music therapy part of their child's program, the positive effects can be transformative.

Physical Therapy (PT)

Physical therapy uses physical exercise and other activities to improve gross motor skills—the large-scale movements of the arms, legs, and torso. PT also helps build strength, balance, coordination, mobility, and endurance. Unfortunately, PT isn't widely offered to autistic chil-dren, partly because autistic children often show strengths in certain aspects of gross motor function, like the ability to walk, run, jump, and climb with ease. But many autistic children have a more limited set of movement patterns—they tend to move their bodies in the same way day-to-day and may not have as many opportunities to expand their movement repertoire. Some avoid sports and other physical activities because participation may lead to sensory overload or because they lack foundational skills in balance and coordination.

Not all physical therapists have the training or experience to sup-port autistic children, but those who do can help children in several important ways, like improving balance, coordination, and control over movement, especially hyperactive, impulsive movements. PT can also help improve hand-eye coordination, body awareness, and physical safety. One of the great benefits of improved gross-motor movement is that it gives a child greater confidence in their ability to successfully navigate a range of environments.

Speech-Language Therapy (SLT)

Speech-language therapy helps people understand language, express themselves through language, produce sounds clearly, use language for social interaction, and develop the oral-motor skills to efficiently chew and swallow. Parents often view SLT as the most important therapy for their child because they're eager to improve their child's communication. As you've learned in this chapter, communication requires a set of foundational sensory, motor, and cognitive skills, so a strong understanding of all developmental domains is important when setting out to build language skills. Speech-language pathologists (SLPs) (also called speech-language therapists) have varying levels of experience and understanding of neurodevelopment in autism. If exploring speech-language services for your child, ask how the therapist supports the sensory, motor, and cognitive precursors for communication, or look for therapists who can provide "co-treatment" sessions or "co-treats." These are sessions where two therapists from different disciplines work together in a session. For example, a speech-language pathologist working together with an occupational, a music, or a physical therapist in your child's therapy sessions could be an effective way to support your child's language development.

SLPs also vary in their training in nonspeech forms of communication, which fall under the umbrella of augmentative and alternative communication (AAC). Reading, writing, and typing for communication are considered forms of AAC, and SLPs differ in their experience, knowledge, and comfort level when it comes to supporting these skills in autistic children.

Counseling

Counseling encompasses a wide range of therapeutic services offered by professionals from many fields, including psychology, marriage-family therapy, social work, and clinical counseling. Within each of these fields, there are many different approaches as well, including cognitive-behavioral therapy, solution-focused therapy, play-based therapy, strength-based therapy, narrative therapy, acceptance and commitment therapy, and many others.

Counseling often takes place through conversations. For children who have the cognitive and language skills to engage with a counselor in this way, there can be great benefits for social-emotional development and overall well-being. When family members receive counseling services to support their own well-being, it can strengthen family relationships and benefit a child's development.

Behavior Therapy

In the next chapter you'll learn how behavior therapy (also known as applied behavior analysis, or ABA) can be part of a neurodevelopmental approach to autism.

The Role of Telehealth Therapies

One of the greatest challenges parents face is the limited availability of professional services in many areas. It may be hard for you to locate professionals who can deliver services in your area, and those you find may have long waitlists. Telehealth therapy services can be a great way to access professional support more quickly and easily. Research shows telehealth therapy can support a child's developmental progress. If your child doesn't engage well with a therapist virtually, telehealth therapy can still be effective as long as you or another caregiver can participate and carry out the recommended strategies. This format—telehealth caregiver coaching—has the added benefit of empowering you with knowledge and skills that you can use with your child anytime you're together in any setting.

Take-Home Message

The services reviewed here are just starting points. Many other therapy services can also be helpful. Great partners can be found in many places. There's no training, degree, or certification that will tell you if a person has the potential to be a great partner for you. But with your understanding of your child's neurodevelopmental profile, you can feel confident evaluating how well any service or professional matches your child's needs.

In the next chapter you'll learn how to get the most out of behavior therapy—one of the most widely available and most recommended services for autism.

Chapter 7

THE HEART OF BEHAVIOR

ABCs and More

Amy, an energetic seven-year-old with red hair and pale blue eyes, was rummaging through the toys in her bedroom closet when she saw an old finger-painting kit.

"Jessica painted with me!" she said, smiling as she pointed to the box.

Her parents looked at each other stunned. Jessica had been Amy's in-home behavior therapist when she was four. Back then she spoke very little and seemed to be in her own world. Her parents never thought she'd remember anything from that time. Jessica was one of eight behavior therapists who worked with Amy between ages two and six. All the therapists had been helpful, but Jessica was truly a blessing. They remembered her as warm, kind, and capable— someone who taught Amy how to get dressed, how to feed herself, and so much more. She brought structure to their home and created stable routines at a time when life often felt chaotic.

Many families like Amy's have wonderful experiences with behavior therapy, also known as applied behavior analysis (ABA), which is the most recommended therapy for autism by doctors and psychologists.

But ABA is also one of the most polarizing topics in autism. Some autistic adults remember their childhood ABA experiences as traumatic. They felt forced to change in ways that didn't align with their sense of self. Some believe ABA devalues autistic differences and imposes neurotypical standards.

Of course, not all approaches to ABA are identical, and fortunately many of the practices used twenty years ago are no longer used today. ABA has evolved so that more programs are using a naturalistic approach, meaning they look for ways to create learning opportunities in children's everyday routines. ABA sessions are often centered on the routines, settings, and play activities that are a natural part of a child's life. More ABA programs are trying to base goals and strategies on knowledge of neurodevelopment and are prioritizing a child's sense of safety and trust, promoting choice, gaining a child's assent, and emphasizing skill building. These are all important steps in the right direction.

Through my studies of neurology, neurodiversity, and behavior, I see that ABA programs can be designed to affirm the principles of neurodiversity and can be tailored to a child's unique neurodevelopmental profile. The overarching purpose of ABA, after all, is to help people do more of the behaviors that serve them well. For your child, it means creating enriching experiences—the kinds of experiences that build confidence, instill joy, and fuel your child's desire to continue expanding their abilities.

If you decide to make ABA part of your child's program, you can get the best of what it offers by building your knowledge of ABA principles, tailoring strategies to your child's unique neurodevelopmental profile, and choosing goals that reflect the principles of neurodiversity.

ABA Basics

ABA comes from a field of psychology called behaviorism, which looks at how a person's surroundings influence their behavior. All behavior originates from brain networks, and brain networks are influenced by factors inside the body and in the environment. In chapter 6 you learned many tools for supporting brain networks "from the inside" by optimizing brain-body health and "from the outside" using the just-right challenge. Now you'll see how ABA principles and practices can further support brain networks "from the outside." When this is done with a child's neurodevelopmental profile in mind, ABA techniques can look a lot like the just-right challenge.

ABC FRAMEWORK

If your child has received ABA services, you're probably already familiar with the ABC model:

ABC Model
A̲ntecedent → *B̲ehavior* → *C̲onsequence*

Antecedents are the things or events that come before a behavior, and consequences are what happen after a behavior. Changing antecedents and consequences are two main approaches ABA uses to change behavior. All the steps you learned about in the last chapter for setting up the just-right challenge fall in the category of antecedents. This is just one of the ways that ABA and other therapeutic approaches overlap.

BRINGING THE BRAIN INTO ABA

What you know about your child's unique neurodevelopmental profile from chapter 6 can guide how you approach making changes to antecedents and consequences. I think of it as bringing the brain into ABA, and it's the approach we use at Cortica.

> *CORTICA'S NEUROBEHAVIORAL FRAMEWORK*
> *(ABBC Model)*
> *Antecedent → Brain → Behavior → Consequence*

In the next three sections of this chapter, you'll learn how to do this for your child by choosing behaviors that matter, setting up for success, and using natural consequences.

Choosing Behaviors That Matter

The principles of neurodiversity should guide your selection of the skills to teach your child. Think first and foremost about which skills will serve your child based on your knowledge of their neurodevelopmental profile. Behaviors that you select should be those that meet the criteria of the just-right challenge. They should not be based on expectations from neurotypical development. Best-selling British author Matt Haig, who has autism and ADHD, says:

> *In the olden days left-handed people were told to hold the pen with their right hand, but they were always left-handed; maybe it's the same with autism. Maybe there's a lot of things where you try to*

be a round peg and you're actually a square peg and that's fine. You just therefore create more square holes.

Many parents agree with this view but feel that until there are more inclusive places in the world for neurodivergent minds, their child should learn how to function in a world designed for neurotypical minds. But forcing neurotypical standards on an autistic mind comes at a cost. The terms *masking* and *camouflaging* refer to the steps autistic people take to blend into social situations where neurodivergence isn't understood or welcomed. It can include behaviors like

- forcing eye contact during conversations
- imitating smiles and other facial expressions
- mimicking gestures
- hiding or minimizing personal interests
- developing a repertoire of rehearsed responses to questions
- scripting conversations
- pushing through intense sensory discomfort, like loud noises
- disguising repetitive behaviors (e.g., replacing preferred behaviors, like flapping hands or spinning, with less obvious ones, like clenching teeth or tapping a foot)

Camouflaging can lead to "autistic burnout," when intense physical, mental, or emotional exhaustion can also be accompanied by a loss of skills. Anxiety and depression are often part of this experience.

You can grow your child's abilities while honoring their autistic identity and supporting their long-term mental health by taking these steps:

1) Teach self-care skills.

2) Extend your child's special interests or "enthusiasms."

3) Make typical social practices optional.

SELF-CARE SKILLS

Self-care includes a wide range of skills that promote any aspect of physical, mental, social, emotional, or spiritual health. Physical self-care skills, like using the bathroom, dressing, and eating meals, are routinely included in ABA programs. And more programs are beginning to include physical exercise during ABA sessions because research studies have found that physical exercise improves developmental skills in autism. Some of the physical activities I've seen children benefit from include walking, jogging, running, hiking, swimming, biking, riding a scooter, weight lifting, CrossFit, rock climbing, paddleboarding, rowing, tennis, and general fitness activities like push-ups, sit-ups, leg lifts, bear crawls, squats, jumping jacks, and jump rope. Introducing your child to a new form of physical exercise often works best with one-to-one instruction from a caregiver, therapist, trainer, or coach. But if your child is already familiar with the activity and enjoys group interactions, you can enroll them in group classes or sports teams. That said, jumping on a trampoline is one form of physical activity to use with caution. Trampoline use requires close supervision to avoid injury. Injuries tend to happen more often in children under the age of six and when multiple people are bouncing together, especially people of different sizes. If your child's use of a trampoline is unstructured, meaning there isn't someone guiding your child to jump at a particular speed or rhythm, then the sensory stimulation they receive may be erratic, and for some children this can be dysregulating.

In addition to goals for physical self-care skills, prioritize self-care skills that support your child's mental health. These are some of the skills I've seen children benefit the most from:

Experiencing nature

Ecotherapy, or nature therapy, is a mental health therapy that involves experiencing nature to improve well-being. It's based in the idea that humans have a deep connection to nature. Research studies have found that spending time outdoors improves mood and promotes relaxation. There are many ways spending time in nature can be part of an ABA program. It can be used as an antecedent strategy to promote regulation and set up your child for success in a task. It can be used as *non-contingent reinforcement*, which is a reward that's given without needing to be earned. Time spent in nature also seems to have added benefits if you're making an effort to notice aspects of the environment, like the details of trees, colors of flowers, or shapes of clouds. Children often enjoy a "nature scavenger hunt," which involves creating a list of different things that your child can find on a hike or other outing in nature.

Listening to or making music

Research studies have found that music activates a broad and diverse set of brain networks, including areas used for sound processing, emotion, memory, and movement. Because of music's profound effects on the brain, it provides a rich medium for building sensory, motor, cognitive, language, social, and emotional skills. Self-care skills related to music could include learning how to access music from different sources (radio, apps, etc.), how to use music-related devices (headphones, stereos, phones, computers, etc.), learning about different types of music, learning to communicate musical interests and preferences with others, and, of course, learning to make music by playing a musical instrument or using digital media.

Observing or creating artwork

Art offers a wealth of opportunities for children to develop new skills. Drawing, painting, and sculpture are just some examples of art forms that provide rich sensory experiences and can be used to develop fine motor skills. Art can also support cognitive, language, and social-emotional development. Art has provided an important route for self-expression for autistic artists, like Stephen Wiltshire, Bryn Graves, Jon Adams, Maxwell Bitton, Megan Rhiannon, Mikaela Sheldt, Jonathan Lerman, and Jeremy Sicile-Kira. If you're not familiar with their work, look them up online to be inspired (see the Guide to Resources at the back of this book for more information).

Preparing food, gardening, caring for animals, writing or journaling, participating in service activities, and mindfulness practices are other self-care skills that have the potential to support your child's mental well-being.

Your child's self-care goals should be personalized to their interests. If your child doesn't tell you or show you what interests them, choose something that you personally enjoyed doing when you were growing up or as an adult. Your firsthand knowledge will help you set your child up for success using prompts and other antecedent strategies that you'll learn later in this chapter.

SPECIAL INTERESTS OR "ENTHUSIASMS"

If your child has a special interest—something they love to think about, talk about, or do—view it as an opportunity to engage and expand their skills. Too often, parents and professionals view special interests as "obsessions" or "restricted interests" and try to discourage them. But special interests are meaningful and serve an important purpose. In her blog, the autistic writer Paige H. N. says, "My special interest was important because it gave me the ability to focus for long periods of time without moving on to something else. My special interest killed any boredom I had; it never got tedious for me. It filled my time when I had nobody to play with as a kid. My special interest meant the whole world."

More and more we're recognizing that special interests can be extended in ways that allow children to grow skills in other areas. An effective way to extend a special interest is to provide opportunities for children with the same interest to meet up and do an activity together. Having a social group structured around a special interest, like Legos, gaming, trivia, music, or other interests, can boost confidence, reduce anxiety, and create a sense of safety. Shared interests are a powerful way to build connection and form peer relationships for all people, whether autistic or neurotypical.

As you think about which behaviors to teach, remember to include your child's special interests and look for ways to expand those interests so they can foster growth in other areas. If those interests change, embrace the new ones and build on them.

Special interests and the self-care skills discussed in the previous section provide abundant opportunities for creating the just-right challenge to advance your child's sensory, motor, cognitive, language, social, and emotional skills. In this way special interests and self-care skills provide an entry point for teaching just about any developmental skill that may be appropriate for your child.

TYPICAL SOCIAL PRACTICES

Connecting with others is important for your child's well-being, but the best way to help your child do this isn't by encouraging or requiring them to follow social customs. Typical social interactions generally include talking while making eye contact and using a variety of facial expressions and hand gestures. Social gatherings and parties also involve tolerating crowds of people. Since your child's preferred way of connecting with others may look quite different, forcing typical social behaviors may be harmful to their social-emotional development and contribute to anxiety, depression, and ultimately burnout. Some examples of neurotypical social customs that are sometimes included in ABA programs include making eye contact, imitating facial expressions, or memorizing rehearsed responses to questions. If you find these goals are part of your child's ABA program, talk with your child's program supervisor about replacing these with self-care skills or goals that extend your child's special interests.

A promising approach to teaching social skills comes from acting classes, participation in theater groups, and other associated activities. I've had the opportunity to work with autistic children and adults who have had positive experiences learning social and communication skills through the dramatic arts. Autistic author Jory Fleming says that taking part in theater allowed him to practice communication as the character he was playing. He found it easier to speak when he was onstage, since spontaneous social interaction wasn't required. He also found he had a knack for memorizing lines and enjoyed being able to speak from the guise of a character.

Autistic actor and Broadway star Mickey Rowe says that as a child he loved to pretend he was a pirate:

> *When you are acting, you always have a clear character. This is why autistic kids often love wearing costumes. . . . It gives them a specific lens with which to interact with the world. It tells them how to behave. . . . Being a pirate made it so that I knew what I was supposed to do in any given moment. I knew how I was supposed to act and what I was supposed to do, because I'd witnessed it being done in movies, in books, and on TV. If I was just Mickey, what was that role? What is Mickey supposed to do in any given situation? I didn't know! I couldn't intuit those things like nonautistic kids. But a pirate? That, I knew. That was a lens I could use.*

Acting allows a person to expand their repertoire for human behavior. Many options become available, and there isn't a single right way to behave. Having the option to move in and out of character can be empowering.

Setting Up for Success

Once you know where to focus your teaching efforts, the next step is to use what ABA therapists call *antecedent strategies* to set your child up for success. Think about a time when someone set *you* up for success. Maybe it was a teacher, a coach, a partner, or a boss. That person understood what you needed to succeed at a task. They laid the groundwork and provided support. Setting someone up for success is one of the kindest, most generous things we can do. It requires knowledge about the person's past experiences and current abilities.

It also requires knowledge of the task itself and what's needed to complete it. If you're thinking this sounds a lot like the just-right challenge, you're right. This is just one of the ways that ABA and occupational therapy use different words to talk about similar things.

From the neurological point of view, it makes sense why setting your child up for success, or creating the just-right challenge, is so important. When we perform a task, the underlying brain networks strengthen. To strengthen the appropriate networks, it's important to perform behaviors in the right ways so that errors don't become hardwired in the brain. This is the rationale for the well-known teaching method called *errorless learning*. Guiding your child to practice new skills without error also allows them to experience success instead of failure. This increases the likelihood they'll be willing to try again in the future. Few things are as rewarding as the experience of success.

You're probably using antecedent strategies throughout the day without giving it a second thought. For example, to help your child do their homework, you might create a clean workspace, provide good lighting, and turn off the TV. To help your child get to sleep, you might read a story, turn on soothing music, and dim the lights. Most of the elements of the sleep improvement plan in chapter 5 are antecedent strategies.

Antecedent strategies also help prevent undesired behaviors. To reduce the chance your child has a meltdown at the grocery store, you might show them your shopping list so they know what items you'll be getting, or if they're sensitive to sound, you might have them put on headphones or earmuffs when entering the store. To make sure your child doesn't run in the store parking lot, you might put your arm on their shoulder, hold their hand, or tell them to stay with you.

When antecedent strategies are used as a direct cue for a behavior, they're called *prompts*. Some examples of prompts are

- guiding your child's hands (physical prompt) (Note that it's important not to force your child's movements, only to guide them. If they resist, try other strategies.)
- saying words, like instructions or encouragement (verbal prompt)
- demonstrating the behavior or showing a picture (visual prompt)

You can use the neurodevelopmental profile you created for your child in chapter 6 to create individualized prompts and other antecedent strategies.

ANTECEDENT STRATEGIES FOR SELF-REGULATION

As you learned in chapter 5, the autonomic nervous system regulates the body's arousal state—the balance between the "fight, flight, freeze" and "rest and digest" states. Strategies to help your child regulate arousal are some of the most important you can provide. From a "just right" arousal state, your child can practice their current skills and learn new ones; from a state of hyper- or hypo-arousal, this is much more difficult.

Strategies that help one person self-regulate may not help another. Consider the way some people focus better with music in the background while others need silence and how some people think best while pacing or fidgeting while others need to be still.

Review what you know about your child in each developmental domain, then review the common antecedent strategies below and circle any that you think will help your child self-regulate.

Sensory-Motor Strategies

The phrase "sensorimotor lifestyle" refers to a daily routine that incorporates many of these strategies on a regular basis to support a child's self-regulation and development.

SOUND

Reducing exposure to sound by using headphones, earplugs, or earmuffs, especially in crowded spaces

Reducing exposure to specific sounds, like vacuums and blenders

Turning on background noise, like a fan or a sound machine that can provide "white noise" (some people prefer lower frequencies, called "brown noise")

Turning on music that's calming for your child

SIGHT

Finding ways to limit visual input, such as putting cardboard dividers on a desk, wearing sunglasses, or wearing a hat

Reducing exposure to fluorescent lights

Dimming the light

Spending time in a space with neutral colors and without clutter

Spending time in a space with bright colors and items that your child finds interesting to look at

TOUCH

Avoiding clothing that your child finds uncomfortable

Letting your child know before you touch them and allowing them to look at where you'll touch them

Giving your child the option to explore objects by touch

SMELL

Avoiding scents that bother your child

Offering your child pleasant natural scents that they enjoy, like scents from flowers, fruits, or essential oils

Offering your child the chance to smell objects or items before using them

BODY AWARENESS

Providing deep-pressure sensory input, like squeezing part of your child's body or giving a firm hug

Using a weighted blanket or weighted vest (use with caution since too much weight or prolonged use can cause injury)

Using a "body sock" or ACE bandage to wrap part of your child's body so they feel resistance when they move

Providing opportunities for "heavy work," such as pushing or pulling heavy objects

Providing opportunities for physical exercise

BALANCE AND MOTION

Providing opportunities to swing in a controlled, rhythmic pattern

Providing opportunities to spin, rock, or roll in a controlled way

Sitting or bouncing on a yoga ball

Providing opportunities for physical exercise

Giving snacks and drinks at regular intervals

Providing ways to cool down or warm up

Using strategies to promote regular bowel movements, such as good hydration, increased fiber intake, and regular physical exercise

Cognitive Strategies

Telling your child what they can expect (offering information about what will happen)

Giving your child a schedule to make events more predictable

Engaging your child in topics they're interested in

Offering puzzles or games your child finds appealing

Giving your child something to remember, or a series of things to remember, and then asking about those things later

Engaging your child's imagination

Giving your child a problem to solve, like a math problem or another problem

Language/Communication Strategies

Using a visual schedule (e.g., creating a written schedule with words and/or pictures)

Reducing spoken language and finding ways to provide information in a visual form (e.g., using written or typed words, pictures, or videos)

Allowing your child to refer back to visual information as needed

Using clear, literal language (e.g., avoiding vague directions or statements with multiple meanings)

Social-Emotional Strategies

Reducing the number of people nearby, especially people your child doesn't know

Including another child in an activity with your child

Using positive "self-talk" (e.g., giving your child statements they can use before a task to encourage themselves, like "I can do this," "I am strong and capable," "I can calm my body," "I can learn new things," "I can try my best"

Ensuring that the people your child interacts with recognize their competence and treat them with genuine respect

USING PROMPTS TO TEACH NEW SKILLS

Prompts are one of the most important techniques you can use to teach your child new skills and to assist them with skills they already have. Prompts are generally categorized into three types:

Physical—guiding your child's hands to complete a movement. If you're moving your child's hands through the entire task, the prompt is called *full*. If you're providing physical guidance for only part of the task, the prompt is called *partial*. Physical prompts use touch, so they give your child tactile sensory input.

Verbal—using words or sounds to help your child carry out a task, like repeating an instruction, giving encouragement, or saying anything else to help your child complete a task. Verbal prompts use spoken words, so they provide your child with auditory sensory input.

Visual—using a picture, written words, or a video or demonstrating the task so that your child can see you do it before they try. A visual prompt that uses a gesture, like pointing, reaching, or nodding, is sometimes called a *gestural* prompt. A visual prompt that involves arranging the position of objects that your child sees is sometimes called a *positional* prompt.

Since prompts involve changing the sensory information your child receives, the information from their neurodevelopmental profile can be very helpful when you decide what prompts to use. For example, if your child processes visual information more easily than auditory information, using a visual prompt might work better. If your child has reduced body awareness, a physical prompt may help bring their awareness to the part of the body they need to move.

When you use prompts, it's a good idea to use the *least intrusive* prompt that allows your child to carry through successfully. Because physical prompts involve physically touching and moving your child's body, they are usually considered the *most intrusive* prompts. These are often needed when you begin teaching a new skill but should be reduced (faded) and removed as soon as your child can do the task without them.

Anytime you decide to use a prompt, also begin thinking about how to remove it. This is called *prompt fading*. This is very important, because if you continue to provide prompts after they're no longer needed, your child will begin to rely on them. The skill can become *prompt-dependent*, which means your child uses the skill only when they get the prompt. In the brain it means the network that performs the behavior has "wired" to the network that receives the prompt. If your child needs a physical prompt when learning a new skill, try to reduce the prompt from full to partial as soon as you can. As your child's skill improves, try to remove the physical prompt and use a verbal or visual prompt instead. Then try fading these prompts as your child's skill continues to improve. As your child's skills grow, you should reduce the support you provide, just as you've learned to do with the just-right challenge.

PREVENTING MELTDOWNS AND TANTRUMS

Meltdowns are episodes of dysregulation that happen when the brain's ability to maintain a regulated state is overwhelmed. You can think of this as a state of *overload*. Sensory information, like sights, sounds, and other sensations, can contribute to overload, especially for children with hypersensitivities. Overload, or feeling overwhelmed, can also happen when your child is given information that they find unsettling, like being told that plans are changing or being asked to do a task that's hard for them. New or unexpected social situations with unpredictable sensory information can also contribute to overload.

Tantrums, on the other hand, are episodes of dysregulation that happen because a child can't have something they want. This may look like a meltdown, but the trigger is different. A meltdown happens because a child is being overloaded by stimuli, and a tantrum happens because a child wants something they don't have.

A meltdown is sometimes called a "bottom up" problem or a problem of the "downstairs brain." This means the problem is coming from the parts of the brain that are processing incoming information. And the cause of the meltdown is the information coming up from the body's senses to the brain. So you can prevent meltdowns by reducing your child's exposure to overwhelming sensory information.

A tantrum, on the other hand, is a "top down" problem or a problem of the "upstairs brain." The part of the brain that makes decisions (prefrontal cortex) initiates the tantrum to get something it wants. If you give in, the prefrontal cortex considers it a win and will repeat this behavior in the future. Once you understand the origin of tantrums and how your actions will influence your child's future behavior, you can see that not responding to a tantrum may very well be an appropriate response. But it's not appropriate for a meltdown. If your child has a meltdown, you should reduce anything that's contributing to their overload and take steps to help them return to a regulated state.

Using Natural Consequences

Natural consequences are the outcomes that happen naturally from what we do. For example, if your child opens a box of raisins, a natural consequence is getting to eat the raisins. If they play keys on a piano, they'll get to hear the sounds of the notes. If they push the power button on the remote control, the TV turns on. These consequences happen naturally without you or anyone else having to do anything.

Consequences are called *reinforcers* if they encourage someone to perform a behavior more often. Getting to eat the raisins, getting to hear notes on the piano, and seeing the TV turn on would all be considered *natural reinforcers* if they lead your child to do the behaviors more in the future. The opposite of a natural reinforcer is an *unrelated reinforcer*. If your child opens a box of raisins, and then you give your child a video game to play, the video game would be an unrelated reinforcer if it leads your child to open more raisin boxes in the future.

Using natural reinforcers with your child is better than using unrelated reinforcers, because natural reinforcers help prepare them for real-world settings where they'll be exposed mainly to natural reinforcement. Unrelated reinforcers may be helpful at the start of your child's ABA program, but in the real world, your child will need to do things because of the natural outcomes that happen from their actions. You or a therapist won't always be there to give a high-five, a piece of candy, or two minutes on a video game as reinforcement for their behavior. Applying new skills to multiple settings, including real-world settings, is called *generalization*. An important goal of ABA is to generalize your child's skills to different people and settings, and using natural reinforcers helps this happen.

The overarching purpose of ABA is to maximize reinforcement—to help people get the outcomes that are meaningful to them and will lead them to do more of the behaviors that serve them well. There are different ways that behaviors can be naturally reinforcing. They can lead to a desired item (like the raisins in the last example) or a desired experience (like hearing piano sounds or watching the TV). They can get someone's attention. Or they can simply feel good.

Here are more examples of natural reinforcers:

- seeing yourself do something better than you did before
- accomplishing something you've been working toward
- carrying out a spiritual or religious ritual that has meaning to you
- carrying out acts of service that benefit others

Laying the groundwork for this type of reinforcement starts early in a child's life. Even before they may show the ability to understand, it's important for them to see others carry out these kinds of behaviors and hear them talk about why they do them. Children need to receive messages about the inherent value of many types of behaviors, starting with basic life skills and expanding to activities in music, arts, athletics, academics, spirituality, and service. This can be as simple as allowing your child to see you doing a variety of activities and talking out loud about

- the reasons why you do them (e.g., for example, why you work at your job, why you go to religious or spiritual services, why you carry out acts of service, why you sing or play a musical instrument, why you make art, why you play a sport, etc.)
- what they mean to you
- how they make you feel
- how what you do helps yourself or others
- where you started and how far you've come

ABA Therapy That Fits Your Family

On your journey you may have come across different ABA approaches to autism. These are some of the most widely used:

Discrete Trial Training (DTT)

Incidental Teaching (IT)

Pivotal Response Treatment/Training (PRT)

Early Start Denver Model (ESDM)

Enhanced Milieu Teaching (EMT)

Reciprocal Imitation Training (RIT)

Improving Parents as Communication Teachers
    (Project ImPACT)

Joint Attention, Symbolic Play, Engagement and Regulation
    (JASPER)

Social Communication, Emotional Regulation, and
    Transactional Support (SCERTS)

Early Achievements

The reason so many different approaches have been developed is that autistic children have different neurodevelopmental profiles, and no single approach meets the needs of all children. Each approach reflects the background of its creators because the approaches are based on their education, clinical experience, research background, and personal perspective. The same is true of Cortica's neurobehavioral approach. It grew out of my own experience as a neurologist and behavior analyst and years of clinical and research collaboration with physicians, psychologists, board-certified behavior analysts (BCBAs), developmental therapists, and counselors.

The challenge in front of you is to choose how ABA fits into the life of your child and family. There are many ways for families to approach this decision. Some need the convenience and affordability of a provider who can start services quickly, can come to the home, and will accept their insurance. Some evaluate multiple providers and choose the one who uses an approach they feel most comfortable with. Some decide to forego ABA services and instead work with therapists who offer relationship-based approaches, like DIRFloortime (DIR = Developmental, Individual Differences, Relationship-Based) or RDI (Relationship Development Intervention). Some live in areas of the country or the world where no ABA services are offered, and they find other ways to support their child (see the Guide to Resources in the back of the book for ideas).

Allow your knowledge of your child and what matters most to your family to guide your decision. If you choose to partner with an ABA provider, participate fully at every opportunity and make the most of what they offer for parent education and coaching. The quality of your participation makes a big difference when it comes to your child's progress in ABA therapy. With your knowledge of ABA principles, your child's neurodevelopmental profile, and the principles of neurodiversity, you can help your child get the most out of all that ABA has to offer.

Chapter 8

A HAPPY, HEALTHY NEST

Nurturing Your Family

In medical school and during my residency, I studied under doctors who'd broken up families. They practiced medicine during the mid-twentieth century, a time when doctors routinely told parents to put their young autistic children in institutions where horrific human rights abuses were later discovered. To think about it is chilling. The weight of past wrongdoings should be a force that fuels us all—professionals, parents, and other members of the autism community—to direct our energy toward supporting families. Thanks to the neurodiversity movement and advances in medical, developmental, behavioral, and mental health services, the future for autistic children and their families is filled with more hope and possibility than ever before.

But it can be hard to feel hopeful when you're facing real struggles every day. There's no doubt that the challenges can make it harder to appreciate what you've already accomplished and make it harder to see what's possible. And the fact is, no matter how much you plan, reality usually looks different.

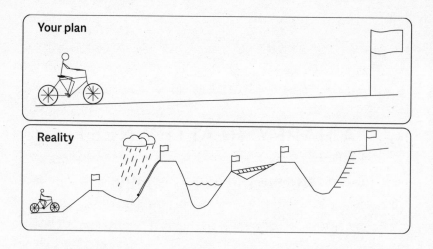

Parents who are going through a particularly tough stretch sometimes ask me, "Will it always be this hard?" The answer is, it doesn't have to be. There are things you can do today to help you get to a better place. Author and activist Anne Lamott says, "Hope begins in the dark, the stubborn hope that if you just show up and try to do the right thing, the dawn will come. You wait and watch and work: you don't give up." No matter what's happening today, there are reasons to be hopeful and steps you can take to create a happy, healthy home for your whole family.

Spreading the Spotlight

Autism and all that comes with it have a way of stealing the spotlight and making everything else fade into the background. As author Kelsey Timmerman wrote after his son Griffin was diagnosed with autism, "So much of our hearts and minds have been wrapped up trying to learn what autism means and what to do and how to feel. . . . Much of whatever free time was left after a day of wiping ends of kids, feeding, bathing, and putting them to bed was spent talking about autism." I see parents pour time, energy, and money into therapies, appointments, and unending to-do lists. On top of this, hours and hours can be consumed by the online rabbit hole, where thousands of interventions claim to help autism. I admire parents' whatever-it-takes attitude. I know that it comes from a place of profound love and devotion. But sometimes the intense focus on your child and on autism can take a toll on you and your other family members. That's why it's so important to adjust the spotlight so that it shines on all family members.

Family means different things to different people, so your family members might be those connected to you by biological ties, by living arrangements, by shared past experiences, or by who truly shows up for you. When you consider how to spread the spotlight, let yourself be guided by any factors that are important to you.

MAKE TIME FOR INDIVIDUAL INTERESTS

Every family member needs to have opportunities to pursue their individual interests. For older children and adults, some of these opportunities should be on their own, apart from your family.

For each family member, make a list of sports, music, arts, hobbies, and anything else that sparks their interest and energy.

NURTURE RELATIONSHIPS IN PAIRS

In addition to each family member needing time to pursue individual interests, your family also has pairs that need time together to nurture their relationship with each other. If you have a partner, the two of you are a pair. Each parent and each child form a different pair; and if you have several children, they can benefit by sibling "pair time," too.

Write down each pair in your family, how they spend time together now, and what else they might enjoy doing together.

RECOGNIZE GROUP DYNAMICS

If your family has three or more members, you'll have a few small groups, or maybe many, each with its own unique dynamic. If you have more than one child, this might be you with your children. If you have a spouse, it might be your spouse with your children—or both of you with one or more of your children. Write down some of the different combinations of family members who spend time together.

Have you noticed how the interactions change depending on who's in the group? One mom, Briana, said that in her family of four, she and her husband could harmoniously spend time with either of their teenage sons, but not both at the same time. When all four of them were together, chaos erupted. Marcus, with autism, and Matthew, with ADHD, always found something to fight about. After a lot of shouting, some threats, and at times physical injuries, everyone left scarred in some way. Just thinking about the four of them together made Briana's stress level skyrocket.

It can be easy to feel like you're failing when you struggle to get along as a family. But in any group, dynamics change depending on who's present, and adding more people to the mix can often make the dynamic less stable. One thing that can help is changing how and when family members spend time together until the friction subsides. As various members start to interact more smoothly, you can be more flexible. For Briana, what helped was limiting most of their family time to pairs or groups of three for a few months while they met with a marriage-family therapist. The therapist used role-play to guide their interactions during common situations when the four of them were together. What they learned in therapy opened new ways for them to enjoy time together as a family at home and in other settings, like restaurants, movie theaters, and recreation centers.

PRIORITIZE YOUR OWN SELF-CARE

As you spread the spotlight from your child to the rest of your family, you might find it's not easy to do this for yourself. If you're like other parents I know, you worry that taking time for yourself means you're not doing everything you should for your child. But this couldn't be further from the truth. Research studies have found that a parent's sense of well-being, empowerment, and engagement are top factors in determining their child's developmental progress. This means improving your own mental and physical health can translate into developmental gains for your child, just as much as any therapies you set up for your child. Deborah Reber, mom of a neurodivergent son and author of *Differently Wired*, says, "Self-care is never selfish." She urges parents to practice *relentless* self-care. That's some of the best advice I've heard, and I try to pass it along to the parents I work with. I even try to follow it myself so that I have more to give to my patients, my teammates at Cortica, and my own family.

Take a moment to make a list of some self-care practices that work for you, and commit to adding one to your schedule this week. Self-care practices can be anything that's good for you that you enjoy, including sports, music, arts, crafts, yoga, meditation, faith-based activities, support groups, counseling, and volunteering.

CONSIDER THE NEEDS OF SIBLINGS

If you have more than one child, it's important to think about how your other child or children experience having an autistic brother or sister.

Of all human relationships, those between siblings usually last the longest, and children who grow up with an autistic sibling can feel a unique bond, as this sister describes:

> She's my sister, I love her, but I don't have the sort of relationship that I have with other people because she can't understand the way I think and probably I can't understand the way she thinks. But I'm totally dedicated to her . . . and want her to have as much fun and enjoyment in life as possible and . . . be happy in herself.

Some children with autistic siblings feel like they don't get enough of their parents' attention and describe being left out of important conversations that affect the whole family. Others describe needing to grow up quickly and having fears about the future:

> I decided I was an adult by the time I was twelve because I was parenting . . . the whole family. I was really scared. . . . I mean many years of sleepless nights worrying what was going to happen to my parents, what would I do about my brother. . . . It would be me that had to look after him.

Research studies of siblings of autistic children have found a range of experiences and outcomes. Some studies found that siblings are more likely to have mental health conditions, like depression and anxiety, but other studies showed that siblings aren't at greater risk for these conditions. In fact, overall, siblings seem to have healthy academic, behavioral, and mental health profiles. They're also more likely to show compassion for neurodivergent people, and their personal experience is often a factor in wanting to pursue a career in health care or education. While the experiences of kids with an autistic brother or sister vary tremendously and are highly individual, research studies have found that having social support makes a positive difference. This means being able to talk about concerns, being connected to others, being part of a community, and feeling acknowledged, included, and informed. Fortunately, the needs of siblings are getting more recognition today than ever before, and many resources are available, including sibling support groups, individual and group counseling, opportunities to participate in therapy sessions with an autistic sibling, books and online blogs written by siblings, and much more (see the Guide to Resources at the back of this book for more information).

Ideas for Starting a Conversation

Children with an autistic sibling have unique experiences, and getting the chance to talk about them is important. Try these conversation starters:

Some kids who have an autistic brother/sister feel _____
_____. Do you ever feel that way?

Fill in the blank with any of these:

- worried that one day they'll have to take care of their brother/sister
- proud of their brother/sister
- embarrassed by their brother/sister
- lonely
- worried about how their friends will respond to their brother/sister

Some brothers or sisters have questions about _____
_____. Do you have questions about that?

Fill in the blank with any of these:

- why their sibling has autism
- what they can do to help

- whether autism can get better
- who will take care of their sibling in the future if something happens to their parents

Family Roots

In Cortica's neurodevelopment framework, a child's family and home are the foundation, or "roots," of their development.

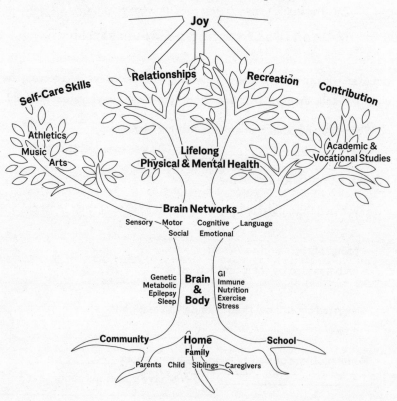

Part of the reason for this is purely practical. There's so much to do—appointments, evaluations, tests, therapy sessions, scheduling, organizing, pickups, drop-offs, and the list goes on and on. All of this is meant to help your child grow into the "branches" of the neuro-development tree, and as you can see, all of this depends in some way on you. If you're energized, hopeful, optimistic, and supported, there's so much you can do. But even the smallest tasks can become overwhelming when you're exhausted, sleep-deprived, anxious, or unsupported.

Another reason why family health and wellness are so important to your child's development is that autistic children are highly influenced by the emotional states of others. As recently as the 2010s, autistic children were mistakenly thought to be "tuned out," but now we know that they often have *heightened* sensitivity to their environment, including other people. And your child is not only affected by the internal state of other family members, but they can also sense when they're in the spotlight by themselves. This can make them feel like their needs require all your attention. No child wants to be a burden, so it's important to make sure everyone in your family gets time in the spotlight, everyone is cared for, and no one is unnecessarily singled out.

When we created our neurodevelopment framework at Cortica, we made sure it applied equally to neurotypical and neurodivergent people—that it captured the important elements of development for all people. Just as you created the neurodevelopmental profile for your child in chapter 1, you can do the same for yourself, your spouse, your other children, and anyone else in your family.

Your Child and You

Shortly after founding Cortica, I hosted a workshop on strengthening the parent-child bond in autism. California's state-funded program for developmental disabilities sponsored the twelve-week workshop, and about sixty parents participated. We met in small groups and talked about topics like how to create a sense of safety and comfort at home by setting up spaces in a particular way, how to give children access to the things they love while also setting necessary limits, and how to handle meltdowns in ways that would strengthen the parent-child bond. We talked about how to create daily schedules to include time for necessary activities, like bathing, dressing, and meals, and also for activities selected and led by a child, like games and other recreation. We discussed how to create safe, comfortable spaces at home where a parent and child could be apart to reset. And we explored many other ways for building understanding and trust between parents and children and creating joyful shared experiences.

Tips for Strengthening the Parent-Child Bond

TIP 1: CREATE SAFE, COMFORTABLE SPACES AT HOME

If your child has hypersensitivities, simplifying the physical environment at home can help reduce their stress level.

- Manage your child's access to electronic devices to avoid overstimulation and do your best to keep electronic devices outside your child's bedroom.
- Keep toys limited to one or two rooms in the house rather than having them spread throughout the house. Keep a small set of toys (between five to ten) in the room and store any others in another space, like a closet, basement, or garage. Rotate the toys from one week to the next so that your child has access to a variety of toys but isn't overstimulated by a cluttered room filled with toys.

- Consider removing items from the home that you don't use and that may contribute to a sense of clutter.
- If your child has their own bedroom, it should be a place where they can be comfortable and safe on their own, without others present. It should be a space where they can engage in any activities they choose as long as these don't pose a risk to safety.

TIP 2: GIVE YOUR CHILD ACCESS TO THE THINGS THEY LOVE, BUT SET APPROPRIATE LIMITS

First, distinguish between what your child *needs* and what they *want*. Examples of needs are using the bathroom, drinking water, eating food (when hungry), and adding or removing clothing (if your child is cold or hot). Examples of wants or desires include electronics, toys, unhealthy snacks, and forms of recreation. Meet your child's needs any time you notice them and when your child makes a request for them.

Proactively give your child the things they desire according to what you feel is appropriate. If they request them more often than what you think is best for them, don't give them access. As you learned in the last chapter, if your child has a tantrum when they don't get something they want, it's important to hold firm and not give in, otherwise the behavior will continue to happen in the future.

TIP 3: TAKE STEPS TO REDUCE THE LIKELIHOOD OF SENSORY OVERLOAD, AND IF MELTDOWNS HAPPEN, TAKE STEPS TO HELP YOUR CHILD RECOVER

As you learned in the last chapter, the best strategy for preventing meltdowns is to reduce your child's exposure to sensory information that can contribute to overload. When a meltdown happens, take steps to reduce anything that's contributing to your child's overload. Help your child return to a regulated state as best you can. Supporting your child in this way strengthens their sense of safety, comfort, and trust.

TIP 4: BALANCE ADULT-LED ACTIVITIES
WITH CHILD-LED ACTIVITIES

Adult-led activities are those in which an adult is guiding your child's behavior. This might be to help your child build skills or engage in certain activities. Many activities in school and therapy sessions are adult-led. Child-led activities are those in which your child guides you or others. Some examples are playing games and other recreational activities. During child-led activities, you allow your child to guide the interaction and you follow their lead. Since so much of your child's day revolves around adult-led activities, it's important to make time for child-led activities. Many parents find this is a great way to end each day.

During our meetings, most of the parents were eager to ask questions and share stories about their children, but not all the parents showed up ready to engage. One soft-spoken mom, Maya, sat back and watched quietly. She didn't say a word in the group sessions, and when I looked her way, she immediately averted her gaze, so I was surprised when she asked if she could schedule an appointment for me to see her four-year-old son.

When I met Ryan, his glasses were tied to the back of his head with a large elastic sports band, and it only took a minute to see why. Ryan ran around my office like he was competing in an obstacle course. He climbed a ladder-back chair, leapt over the coffee table, bounced on and off the couch, and rolled under the desk. Maya sat very still, with her arms crossed, as though she was protecting herself against the overstimulation that his behavior was causing her.

I learned that the day-to-day challenges were extreme. Ryan's dad, Sean, traveled often for work, and since Ryan and his two-year-old brother were both at home, Maya was caring for them 24/7. She told me, "I'm always worried Ryan's going to have a meltdown. He screams, throws things, and even hits me." She shook her head. "I'm on edge even when things are going okay. I think I'm failing as a mom. I love Ryan, but if I'm honest, I don't think I like him." On top of this, she and Sean had decided not to tell any of their family, who all lived outside the country, about Ryan's diagnosis.

Step-by-step we began to work through each component of Ryan's care. We did the appropriate medical tests and started ABA, occupational therapy, speech-language therapy, and music therapy. As the months passed, Ryan made steady progress. His sensory processing abilities improved and his hyperactivity reduced. But even as he made strides and it became clear that he'd soon be ready to enter a general education kindergarten class, Maya remained anxious, had difficulty sleeping, and didn't seem to be encouraged even though Ryan was doing well.

I told Maya and Sean about the social workers and marriage-family therapists in my clinic that they could meet individually, as a couple, or with the entire family. They agreed that it could be helpful and said they'd be willing to give it a try. But when my staff reached out to schedule the appointment, they said no. Unfortunately, this happens a lot, and I understand why. Many people are reluctant to seek mental health services. The idea of counseling—or psychotherapy—can be scary. Talking about emotions and relationships can make some people feel exposed and stir up feelings of vulnerability. But having professional support for mental health is incredibly important. We know from research studies that about one in three moms and one in five dads of autistic children experience depression or anxiety. In today's world I think every person can benefit from mental health support, whether or not depression, anxiety, or autism is part of the equation. Everyone has the potential to experience peace and well-being, because the human brain has this capacity. But it often takes help from others for us to experience these natural states.

When parents decline professional counseling, I look for other options. At one of our visits, I learned that at one time Maya belonged to a community group called Living Well that hosted events for meditation, yoga, and breathwork, but she hadn't participated since Ryan's diagnosis two years ago. So I picked up my prescription pad and wrote, "Living Well: Attend one event per month for one year. Unlimited refills."

She laughed, but it worked. She not only reconnected with the group, but she also invited other parents she'd met at Cortica to join. Sean, inspired by Maya's change, returned to his community soccer league. A few months later they shared Ryan's diagnosis with their extended family and reopened those channels of support. I knew that getting Maya and Sean back into practices that nurtured them was one of the best things I could do for Ryan. Parents sometimes think their autistic child needs to change before things can change for the rest of the family, but the most meaningful and long-lasting changes happen in the family first.

Finding Helpers

Part of the steep learning curve that comes with an autism diagnosis is learning about the wide array of available resources. Having many resources to choose from is far better than the lack of resources parents struggled with just a few decades ago, but it can be hard to tease out the signal from the noise. To navigate the learning curve, it's helpful to have professional partners who can help you focus on what's most important for your family, guide you toward quality interventions, and help you steer clear of others.

When finding your helpers, look for professionals, family members, friends, neighbors, and others who, as Dr. Barry Prizant says, "get it." These are people who recognize that your child and your family are the experts in your own lives. They are people who have the qualities of empathy, flexibility, sensitivity, and humor. They don't try to control you or your child, and instead focus on building positive relationships based on trust. They see your child's behavior as *human* behavior instead of attributing every behavior to autism.

We all need helpers. There's little in life that we can do alone and so much we can do when we access the support, knowledge, experience, and wisdom of others.

The Good Stuff

Autism can be a portal to greater connection, purpose, hope, and joy. Not through any pill, diet, supplement, device, or even autism therapy program (although there are professionals who *can* be a great help). Getting to the good stuff—what at the end of the day makes life truly worth living—happens in another way, one that takes most parents by surprise. It happens through understanding and developing your *family culture*.

The word *culture* is often misunderstood and thought of as referring only to ethnicity or nationality. But culture has a much broader meaning that includes the values, beliefs, and practices that any group of people have in common. Culture includes shared knowledge, assumptions, and what's viewed as right or wrong. Culture determines how we make sense of the world and our place in it.

A few years after Cortica opened its doors, we knew it would be important to define our culture so we could ensure that as we grew to more locations, every Cortica site would embody the values most important to us, like embracing neurodiversity; championing whole-child, family-centered care; and recognizing competence in all our clients, their family members, and our teammates. We used an approach to understanding and defining organizational culture that's been used by other mission-driven organizations, and it's an approach you can use for your own family.

We created

- a vision statement of our overarching purpose
- a mission statement of what we would do day-to-day to get closer to achieving our vision
- a set of values around how we engage with each other and with the families we serve.

....

Cortica's Culture

VISION STATEMENT

To unlock more joy for neurodivergent children and their families every day.

MISSION STATEMENT

To design and deliver life-changing care, one child, one family, one community at a time.

We see possibility. Growth and learning are possible for all. Where others see limits, we see potential.

We get better every day. Excellence is earned through growth and innovation. As teams and as individuals, we seek opportunities to continuously expand our knowledge and improve our abilities.

We care. A lot. We are committed to improving lives. Passion and dedication show through how we take care of the families we serve and the world we share.

We do what's right even when it's hard. Professional ethics and clinical excellence guide all our actions. Integrity means living by our shared values.

We're better together. Collaboration and teamwork are at the heart of everything we do. Our comprehensive model values the contributions of each discipline, as we know our whole is greater than the sum of our parts.

We take care of ourselves and each other. We are compassionate with our clients, our teammates, and ourselves. We value the health of mind, body, and spirit.

We laugh, we cry, we keep it real. Authenticity and humility matter to us. By building relationships based on trust, we create a safe space for everyone.

We enjoy the journey. We have perspective that our mission is not easy. We appreciate both the ups and downs. Our resilience comes from the importance of our mission and the support of our team.

We're all about family. Family wellness is important to us. We nurture client families, our own families, and the Cortica family.

We love what we do. Our work is a calling.

. . . .

If you like the idea of writing a vision statement, a mission statement, and a set of values for your own family, take a moment to complete the questions and statements below. If doing this seems strange, silly, corny, or "out there," I encourage you to do it anyway. You don't have to show it to anyone (but once you've done it, I think there's a good chance you'll want to share it with your family). You may even want to try doing this activity together with your family, or you can try it out on your own first and then bring in other family members.

. . . .

YOUR FAMILY'S VISION: THE "WHY"

What matters most to your family, and why?

What's your purpose as a family, and why?

The reason we're here is to _____.

(Once you've responded to these questions, ask yourself why one more time—this can help you get to a deeper statement of your purpose.)

YOUR FAMILY'S MISSION: THE "WHAT"

What do you and others in your family do that help you achieve your purpose?

What actions have you taken or do you plan to take to make your vision a reality?

How do you interact with each other?

How do your actions reflect what's important to you?

The visionary leader and educator Peter Drucker has said, "Culture eats strategy for breakfast." This popular saying means that culture is more important than strategy (or plan of action)—in other words, having a strong understanding of your purpose and values and acting in harmony with them matters the most for achieving your goals. Any plan you create, any action you take, should reflect your family culture. For example, if what matters most to your family is your connection with each other, but you're not creating opportunities to strengthen those connections (like doing enjoyable activities together), it will be harder to achieve what's important to you. If what matters most is the health and well-being of each family member, then making time for self-care will help you achieve the vision you have for your family.

Even though culture doesn't refer only to ethnicity or nationality, these often have a strong influence on family culture. Your family might have customs or traditions related to your ethnic background, the country or countries of your family's origin, or the country where you now live. You may be part of communities that shape your beliefs and actions, whether they are your neighborhood, your child's school, or online communities that you've chosen to join. Beliefs related to religion, faith, and spirituality play an important role for many people. Any of these and many others may influence your family's culture and may offer you connection, meaning, and purpose.

Identity Wheel

Your family culture is influenced by the identity of each family member. An identity wheel is a way to learn more about each person, how they think about their identity, and what's important to them. If you think your family would enjoy this activity, set aside some time when you can complete these identity wheels and share them with each other.

SOCIAL IDENTITY WHEEL

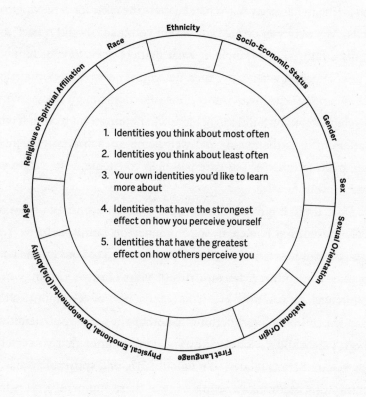

1. Identities you think about most often
2. Identities you think about least often
3. Your own identities you'd like to learn more about
4. Identities that have the strongest effect on how you perceive yourself
5. Identities that have the greatest effect on how others perceive you

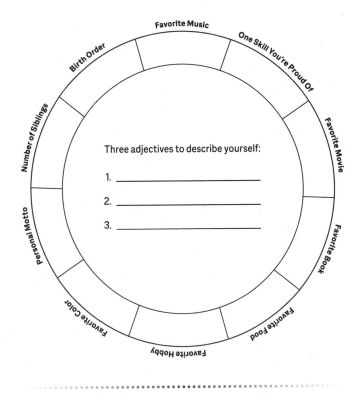

Sometimes physical illnesses or mental health conditions in family members influence family priorities. Knowing about these can help ensure everyone gets the medical care and support they need. For example, moms of autistic children are more likely to have autoimmune conditions, like rheumatoid arthritis and thyroid disease. About one-third of siblings of autistic children have a mental health or developmental diagnosis, like autism, ADHD, learning disability, anxiety, behavior disorder, or mood disorder (like depression). Here are some practices that can be especially helpful if you're navigating health conditions in multiple family members:

- Approach new challenges as a family.
- Take things one day at a time.
- Celebrate small wins.
- Believe in the potential of each family member to continue to learn and grow.

In the next chapter you'll expand your thinking beyond the home to your child's experiences at school and in the wider community. For many children, community activities provide the spark that ignites passion and purpose. You'll learn how to create these kinds of experiences for your child at school and in the community.

Chapter 9

COMMUNITY ADVENTURES

Expanding Your Child's World

Life is either a daring adventure or nothing.

—Helen Keller

Andrew, a sixteen-year-old with autism, ADHD, and epilepsy, just had the best summer of his life.

His days started with a two-mile jog to a café near his home. He was usually the first customer of the day, and the staff greeted him by name. At the start of the summer, his brother or home aide accompanied him, but soon he was going on his own. In the afternoon he often went to the gym with his dad, where he learned to use weight machines for circuit training. He also joined an acting program for autistic youth hosted by a local theater group and was cast in a play with a mix of neurotypical and autistic actors. He was proud to be an actor, and to prepare for the public performance in the fall, he practiced his lines every day.

Andrew also took two trips over the summer. For his sister's wedding, he flew with his family to Mexico for a weeklong stay. Leading up to the trip, his parents had been nervous because family vacations had not gone well in the past. The last attempt two years earlier led to a late-night emergency room visit after a meltdown when he broke his ankle kicking the rental-car door. But Andrew wanted to attend his sister's wedding, and his whole family wanted him to be there, too, so they began planning months ahead. They created a photo book with a story so that Andrew would know what to expect during the trip. They planned daily physical exercise to start each day, and Andrew had a backpack on hand with all the sensory supplies that helped him self-regulate, like headphones, his favorite music, sunglasses, and fidgets. The trip went even better than they'd hoped it would go, and I got to see this for myself in the family wedding photos that showed Andrew beaming.

During the last two weeks of summer, he and his family attended an adaptive outdoor sports and recreation camp, where they hiked mountain trails, biked, kayaked, rode horses, and went rock climbing. On the last day, Andrew told his parents, "I'm going to work here when I'm done with school, and you can come visit me!" His mom told me, "The summer changed all of us. I've never seen Andrew so happy. It was amazing, really. It was life-changing."

While creating experiences in the community for an autistic child or teen can take effort and planning, the rewards that come from these efforts can be incredible—not just for your child but for your whole family. Many autistic adults look back at community activities like sports, recreation, music, arts, camps, and travel as the most positive experiences of their childhood. And these experiences can inspire future pursuits, like influencing your child's eventual choice of work or planting the seeds for lifelong hobbies and other passions. Because having good experiences outside the home is so important for your child, learning how to craft these experiences with appropriate support so your child can succeed is well worth your time.

It's not always possible to find activities or groups that offer a good person-environment fit, and if that's the case for you, see if you can find community partners to help you create them. With the rise of the neurodiversity movement, more people and organizations in communities across the world are dedicated to building inclusive environments. With the right knowledge and support, you can create positive experiences that expand your child's world in exciting new directions.

Choosing a School

School makes up the biggest part of the day for most children and can set the tone for your child's overall mood and behavior. The best school program for your child will depend on their unique neurodevelopmental profile. There's no single right approach for all children, so keep an open mind as you explore the different options available to you.

The main types are public school, private school, and homeschool, and within these categories there are different options depending on your community and school district. When you're considering what will work best for your child, talk with other parents in your area who've been through the process. Even if your child's needs are different from theirs, you'll be able to learn a lot by hearing about their experiences. Consulting with a special education advocate or special education attorney can be helpful, too, if you find you need more in-depth guidance.

PUBLIC SCHOOL

By law, public schools in the United States are required to provide a "free appropriate public education" to students with disabilities. The Individuals with Disabilities Education Act (IDEA) became law in 1975 and requires public schools to provide students with an educational program that's individualized to the students' needs. Before IDEA, public schools routinely turned away students with disabilities; but under IDEA, public schools are required to offer an individualized education program (IEP) with specialized instruction and related services to children with a qualifying diagnosis, like autism.

It's important to know that an *appropriate* education doesn't mean an *optimal* education. Federal law doesn't require public school programs to maximize your child's progress. Many factors influence how much your child's school district will be able to provide, like the level of available funding and the knowledge and experience of the staff.

In public schools the main classroom settings are general education classrooms—often called gen ed or inclusive settings—and self-contained special education classrooms, or special ed. Because IDEA requires school districts to provide children with the "least restrictive environment," districts will first consider whether a gen ed classroom with a standard academic curriculum among neurotypical peers could be appropriate for your child. Your district might be able to provide a one-to-one aide, an adapted curriculum, or other accommodations to support your child in a gen ed classroom.

The other option is a special education classroom. Some special ed classrooms include only autistic students, and others have a wider range of students with different physical or developmental diagnoses. These classrooms usually have fewer students than gen ed classrooms, which can be beneficial for some children. Schools may also offer programs where a child spends time in both gen ed and special ed settings. Some programs include time spent in a "resource room" where a child receives more tailored instruction with a special ed teacher one-on-one or in a small group.

Many communities also have charter schools, which are publicly funded alternatives to typical public schools. These schools are established by teachers, parents, or other members of the community and often adopt a specific educational philosophy or approach, like project-based learning, Montessori education, or others. For many autistic children, charter schools provide a great way to access free public education that may offer better support for their unique sensory, cognitive, or social-emotional needs.

PRIVATE SCHOOL

Private schools fall into two categories: typical and specialized.

Typical private schools mainly serve a neurotypical student population, but some enroll neurodivergent students when they feel they can meet the student's needs. Typical private schools offer a gen ed experience, often with smaller class sizes than public schools, and many provide a broader set of enrichment experiences. Some allow a one-to-one aide in the classroom if they're hired and paid for by you or by an external funding source. For example, a behavior therapist funded by a child's health insurance might be able to support your child in a private school classroom.

"Kind Work"
Instead of Homework

Tanya and Joe, parents of second-grader Laura, enrolled her in a typical private school with a strong focus on children's social-emotional development. This was a great match for Laura, whose cognitive and language skills were advanced for her age, but who needed more support interacting with other children and regulating her emotions.

Tanya and Joe were delighted to learn that instead of having homework, the teacher and students worked together to come up with ideas for "kind work." They'd complete kind-work assignments, some during school and some outside of school, like helping each other with classwork, caring for class pets, and expressing encouragement and appreciation. I learned about this when one day I received a thank-you card from Laura out of the blue. Tanya told me the thank-you card was a kind-work assignment, and Laura had chosen to write the card to me. That made my day!

The school also offered enhanced physical education, including on-site swimming lessons, dance classes, and martial arts. It even had a theater program and an acting instructor, who taught Laura and her classmates how to interpret and express emotions through movements.

After hearing about the school and seeing Laura's progress, I asked Joe and Tanya how they chose the school so that I could share their tips with other parents.

"They chose us," Tanya said. She explained that when they decided to give private schools a try, they weren't sure how to decide between schools, so they applied to the four that were closest to their home. She said, "Only one school invited us for an interview. The admissions officer told us all about their philosophy and their programs and told us she really believed they could give Laura a great education. Honestly, it almost sounded too good to be true." She laughed. "But she was right!"

Specialized private schools are designed specifically for special education. These schools offer small class sizes and may even provide one-to-one instruction. Some specialized private schools serve a broad range of children with special needs, and others focus exclusively on autism. Some specialized private schools for autistic children are dedicated to serving children with specific types of needs. For example, some serve children with high support needs, like children with limited speech, higher levels of repetitive behaviors, and difficulty with self-regulation. Others serve children with low or moderate support needs.

Thriving in a Specialized Private School

Nine-year-old Ella, with autism, ADHD, and a genetic syndrome, spent most of her day in a public school gen ed classroom with thirty students. She also spent one hour each day in a resource room with a special ed teacher and three other students. In gen ed she sat quietly at her desk, looking out the window. She didn't follow the teacher's instructions, complete assignments, or participate in class discussions. But in the resource room her teacher was able to keep her engaged, and she was able to easily do the same assignments she struggled with in gen ed.

Because Ella learned so well in the resource room, her parents wanted to find a specialized private school where she could have instruction like that all day. While they were exploring their options, they asked if we could try medications to help Ella focus. We tried four different medications over three months and none seemed to help.

What *did* help was getting Ella enrolled in a specialized private school with a class of six students, a special ed teacher, and an aide. She participated much better but still had some trouble focusing. After a month, we restarted one of the medications to help her with attention, and her parents and teacher noticed a big improvement. For Ella, the benefits of the medication were not enough to overcome the challenges posed by the gen ed school environment, but once she was in a better school setting, the medication made a clear difference.

HOMESCHOOL

Homeschooling isn't what you might think. Many parents assume it means they'll be responsible for teaching their child, and for that reason, many rule it out right from the start. But homeschooling can be done in a variety of different ways and offers the greatest opportunity for customizing your child's educational program. And it's not something you have to do alone—homeschooling can and should involve a team approach. Your team may include one or more therapists, tutors, learning specialists, teachers, aides, or other professionals or caregivers. One of the main benefits of a homeschool program is flexibility, because you and your team can design the curriculum and schedule. But this flexibility usually does come with greater responsibility, greater investment of time and energy, and potentially greater cost. When you're already facing a busy schedule and many challenges, you might not feel it's possible to take on something like this. But I've seen times when a child's struggles were due to negative experiences in a gen ed or special ed environment, and even though homeschooling took additional effort, it made many of the other struggles go away, and overall life became better for the whole family. Many families try public or private school options first, but if you find your child's needs aren't being met, you may want to explore homeschooling as an option.

An Innovative Hybrid Program

Patrick, a nonspeaking twelve-year-old with autism and ADHD, attended a public middle school in a special ed class with nine other autistic children, all with very high support needs. The teacher and four aides were well trained to support children with aggressive behavior, but Patrick's behavior was more than they could safely manage. The school staff recognized that they couldn't meet Patrick's needs in a public school setting, so they agreed to fund his placement at a private specialized school that had the best track record in the county for helping autistic children with aggressive or self-injurious behaviors. But even at that school, the staff felt unable to support Patrick, and he continued to have episodes of severe behavior that caused injury to himself, other students, and school staff.

The only setting where he seemed comfortable and learned new skills was in a therapy center, where he received one-to-one behavioral and developmental therapies. So his parents asked the school district to fund a unique hybrid program where he would spend mornings receiving one-to-one therapy services at the center and afternoons at his local public middle school with an ABA therapist as his aide. The school district had never supported a program like this, but fortunately they were willing to give it a try.

Patrick thrived with this program. Within a month he was able to participate in gen ed classes at his public middle school for physical education and art and to eat lunch at school, all with the support of his ABA therapist, who was able to carry over effective strategies from the center to the school. This arrangement worked so well for Patrick that he was able to explore new activities, like skiing, trail running, mountain biking, open-water swimming, and eating at restaurants. When parents, school administrators, and community professionals collaborate in innovative ways with a child's best interest in mind, great things can happen.

Person-Environment Fit

Since a strengths-based approach to education relies on creating a good person-environment fit, your child's neurodevelopmental profile (from chapter 6) should guide you when evaluating how well various school environments may meet their sensory, motor, cognitive, language, social, and emotional needs. Your child's sensory profile is especially important, because if the sights, sounds, and smells of the school setting put them into a dysregulated, high-stress state, they'll have a harder time focusing on what's being taught in class.

Because federal law (IDEA) requires school districts to place students in the least restrictive environment, schools place children in gen ed settings whenever possible. But when we consider the person-environment fit, it's clear that we need to think more carefully about what makes an environment restrictive. For example, an environment that feels unsafe, unwelcoming, or, worse yet, threatening can severely restrict your child's emotional development and well-being. When we think about it this way, we recognize that gen ed settings might be extremely restrictive for some children. The ultimate goal should be to change gen ed environments to accommodate the needs of neurodivergent students, but at present the barriers to doing this are high.

When my six-year-old patient Wes started having meltdowns at school and was becoming more withdrawn at home, I went to his public elementary school to observe his first-grade gen ed classroom. When I arrived, Wes was outside on the playground, and what I saw made my heart sink. A child much bigger and older than Wes was following him and aggressively poking him in the back. There were no adults nearby to see what was going on. When I shared this information with his parents, they decided to transfer Wes to a public Montessori charter school that offered a higher ratio of teachers to students, a flexible and individualized curriculum, and a culture of appreciation of diversity. In this setting, Wes thrived.

Social growth happens when your child has the opportunity for consistent and meaningful social interaction, can share mutual interests with peers, and has the chance to deepen relationships over time. Merely being surrounded by other children doesn't ensure social growth and can be socially restrictive if the setting isn't a good fit. If your child's school environment doesn't offer opportunities for social growth, consider exploring other school options or look for ways to create social opportunities outside of school.

Advocates and Attorneys

Special education advocates and special education attorneys can provide a range of services, like recommending schools and other service providers, reviewing IEPs, communicating and negotiating with schools on your behalf, and accompanying you to school meetings. Special education advocates aren't required to have a license or certification, but many have degrees or experience working in special education. Special education attorneys provide many of the same services as advocates and can also prepare legal documents and represent you in legal proceedings if the need arises. Services provided by an advocate are generally less expensive than those provided by an attorney, and school districts are usually more receptive to working with an advocate.

Starting the IEP Process

Becoming well informed is an important step toward getting your child the educational opportunities they deserve. Fortunately, there are many wonderful resources available, including free online resources (see understood.org). Other parents of autistic children who are willing to share their experiences can also be a great resource, and they may have experience working with advocates or attorneys in your area.

To request an evaluation with your school district to see if your child is eligible for an IEP, contact your school and speak to a special education program specialist, or submit a request in writing to a member of the school staff.

School-Provided Evaluations and Therapies

School-provided evaluations and therapies differ in important ways from services offered by other professionals. Knowing these differences can help you understand what to expect from your school district and help you decide whether you need to pursue additional evaluations or services.

For example, psychoeducational assessments conducted by school psychologists generally cover a smaller set of skills than developmental assessments by psychologists in private clinics. If you disagree with the results of a school-provided evaluation, you can request that the school district pay for an independent educational evaluation (IEE) by a psychologist outside of the school district.

The role of therapists in the school setting is often different from their counterparts who practice in private centers or clinics. For example, the role of a school's occupational therapist (OT) is different from the role of an occupational therapist who provides services in a private center or clinic. In schools, the OT's role is to recommend accommodations and supports that help improve a child's performance at school. In comparison, an OT in a clinic setting looks more broadly at sensory processing differences, fine motor skills, self-regulation, and social-emotional development and offers strategies to support a child across multiple settings, not only in school. Direct one-to-one OT services are routinely part of clinic-based programs but are less common in schools. Similarly, speech-language therapy services in schools usually address a smaller range of goals related specifically to your child's educational program. One-to-one school aides provided by a school district come with a range of different experiences and backgrounds and may or may not have training related to autism or child development.

Community and Belonging

In our neurodevelopment framework, your child's experiences at school and in the broader community are foundational to their development, just like their experiences at home—they're the "roots" of your child's development.

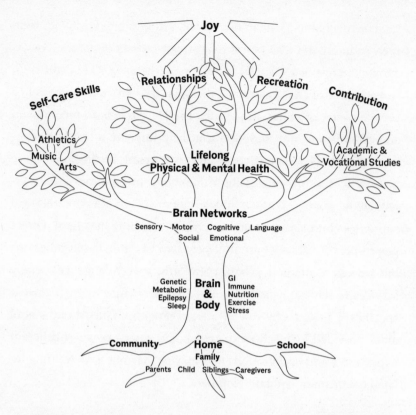

Children of all ages and developmental profiles can have positive experiences in the community. The key is to choose these experiences based on your child's neurodevelopmental profile and then take steps to prepare your child and to prepare others who will take part, including any community partners who will be involved, like class instructors, coaches, program directors, and facility staff. Without these preparations, there's a greater chance that the experience will turn south, which can discourage you from trying again. So start gradually—don't be too ambitious. And as you see your child's response, make changes. You don't have to do it all at once. If you've started down a path and it's not going well, take a break and try again later or move on to something else.

Be open when providing information about your child to potential community partners. If they don't feel their program can meet your child's needs, try to understand why and see if they're open to modifying their program to fit your child's needs. If not, move on to look for others who can.

Throughout this book you've heard about community activities and the benefits they can bring. As with any activity your child does at home, in school, or in a therapy clinic, they're more likely to succeed when the combined challenge—across sensory, motor, cognitive, language, social, and emotional domains—is manageable for them. Some community activities, like athletics, will pose new motor challenges for your child. Learning new motor skills in a one-to-one or small-group setting often works better because this removes the sensory and social challenges that come when surrounded by a large group of children.

Here's a list of activities I've seen autistic children succeed in and guidelines on how to set your child up for success.

Athletics
- Walking, jogging, running, or a combination of these
  - Start with a distance and pace that's comfortable for your child.
  - Many children like to know the goal, so show your child what you're asking them to do by using a timer (e.g., show them how long the activity will last), a step counter (e.g., show them how many steps you'd like them to take), or map (e.g., give them a sense of the route and how long it is).
  - Pick an outdoor setting, if possible.
  - If your child enjoys music, you can consider allowing them to listen to music while exercising.

- Show your child a video on YouTube of people running a race. This can give your child a sense of what they can work toward.
- Involve other people, or have your child join a group if you feel your child will be motivated by doing the activity with others.
- Many children are motivated by seeing their own progress. There are a variety of ways you can create a visual record of their progress, like simply writing down what they do each day in a notebook or on a calendar or using a spreadsheet and creating a graph.
- Hiking
  - Since this involves going out on a trail, make sure you're prepared for any challenges that might come up. Bring another person with you if needed. Pick a trail that you know well and start with a short outing. Gradually increase the distance and difficulty as your child's skills grow.
- Swimming
  - Autistic children often love swimming because they enjoy the sensory experience of being in water. Swimming lessons are a great way for your child to learn basic water safety skills and different strokes, like freestyle and backstroke. Unstructured play in a swimming pool is a good leisure activity, but your child will get more out of swimming if they learn to coordinate their movements using strokes to move through water.
- Bike riding
- Hippotherapy or horseback riding
- Rock climbing
  - Indoor rock-climbing gyms often have times of day when

they're mostly empty. A quiet environment with fewer people is better for many children who are just starting out. Having one-to-one instruction can also help when getting started.

- Martial arts
  - This is often one of the first activities parents think of when their child has difficulties with attention and regulation. It works well for some children but not for all, so if your child doesn't seem to be benefiting, it's worth exploring other activities.
- Gymnastics
- Parkour
- Weight lifting, CrossFit, or personal training
  - These activities can be great for adolescents and young adults.
- Tennis, pickleball, table tennis, badminton, or other racquet sports
  - These activities require a high level of hand-eye coordination (or visual-motor integration). Occupational therapy and physical therapy can help build the prerequisite skills for these kinds of activities.
- Basketball, soccer, baseball, volleyball, or other team sports
  - Team sports like these require a high level of sensory, motor, cognitive, language, and social-emotional skill. If joining a team poses too great a challenge for your child based on their current neurodevelopmental profile, they can still benefit from these activities in modified forms, like one-to-one instruction or small groups. I've seen many children who start with one-to-one instruction become able to join competitive sports teams as their skills grow.

Arts and music

- Voice, piano, or other musical instruments
- Dance
- Dramatic arts (theater, acting, comedy)

Religious or spiritual activities

- Many religious and spiritual communities offer educational and social opportunities for children. If a group experience isn't a good fit for your child, consider individualized ways to nurture your child's development in this area, like hearing stories; reading books; watching shows, videos, or films; or having one-to-one instruction with you or another person with knowledge and experience to share.

Service activities

- It can be powerful for your child to recognize they have the ability to help other people, animals, and the planet, and research studies show that volunteering has a wide range of physical and mental health benefits.

Nature activities

- Farming
- Gardening
- Caring for animals
- Camping

Social groups

- There are many ways to create social group experiences for your child.
  - Include another child (neurodivergent or neurotypical) in your child's therapy sessions.

- Join a social skills group facilitated by a therapist or teacher.
- Find opportunities for your child to engage in activities they enjoy in a group setting.

Outings to public venues like restaurants, shops, theaters, theme parks, museums, sporting events, etc.

- Your knowledge of your child's neurodevelopment—especially their sensory profile—should guide your selection of outings. Be guided by what you *know* they can manage, not by what you *hope* they can manage.
- Planning ahead is essential to success. Prepare by providing your child with stories that tell them what to expect, ensuring adequate sensory supports, and having a backup plan in case things don't go well.

Whatever your child's age or neurodevelopmental profile, they can have positive experiences in the community with preparation and support. If you try something and it doesn't go well, learn what you can from the experience, decide what you'll do differently next time, talk to professional partners or others you trust for guidance, and then try again. Most important, be kind to yourself and recognize that even when things don't go as planned, you're taking on challenges and trying to create enriching experiences for your child. You should feel great about that.

Part 3

LASTING CHANGE

Chapter 10

FINDING WISDOM

Lead with the Spirit, the Mind Will Follow

Peace and joy . . . are every person's birthright.

—Thich Nhat Hanh, spiritual leader and activist

Autism can bring exhilarating moments when you least expect them. For five-year-old Emma's mom, it happened one night while cuddling at bedtime when Emma said her first "I love you." For six-year-old Noah's dad, it happened when he heard Noah reciting passages from *Diary of a Wimpy Kid* and discovered that Noah, who rarely spoke, could read books. For fourteen-year-old Rafael, it was crossing the finish line of his first 10K race; and for twenty-year-old Jordan, the sale of his first painting. For Michael McCreary, the moment came during his first stand-up comedy performance, when he realized he'd found his calling. Every day autistic children and adults discover new abilities, extend their passions, and brighten our world.

But as you probably know all too well, autism can also bring some of the most difficult—at times heartbreaking—moments. Your world can come to a halt if your child stops speaking and you don't know if or when they'll speak again. Seeing your child engage in behaviors that cause harm to them can be agonizing. Even finding places where your autistic child can be fully themselves can feel like a never-ending challenge. Autism magnifies life's everyday ups and downs and demands greater courage, strength, and determination from autistic people and those who love them.

The whole-child path you've been learning about in this book and its five key elements—brain-body health, development, behavior, family, and community—offer a way to recognize and nurture your child's gifts and abilities through even the most difficult times. By seeing your child as multidimensional, intelligent, strong, and whole, you create the space for their gifts to grow and their spirit to flourish, even when obstacles and challenges seem overwhelming.

Here are just some of the gifts I've seen parents recognize and nurture in their children on the whole-child path:

Perseverance
Enthusiasm
Laughter
Honesty
Energy
Intelligence
Exceptional memory
Finding simple joys
Bringing happiness to others
Bringing out patience and compassion in others
Great sense of humor and a knack for making others laugh
Love of sports
Love of music
Passion for figuring out how things work

Valuing friendships and family relationships

Being loving and lovable

Desire to give back to others

Extraordinary abilities like these can be the foundation for meaningful pursuits in the wider world. So it's not surprising that autistic people are involved in nearly every field of work and study. Autistic professionals include scientists, professors, doctors, entrepreneurs, athletes, musicians, writers, reporters, actors, artists, inspirational speakers, CEOs, investors, philanthropists, public officials, chefs, and religious and spiritual leaders. Apart from work, autistic people flourish in an even wider variety of pursuits, including forming meaningful relationships and being mothers, fathers, spouses, caregivers, and friends. So an autism diagnosis is no reason to give up dreams for a future brimming with activity, connection, purpose, and joy. If your child isn't successful with the first things they try, it may help to remember that nobody takes to everything they pursue, whether they're neurotypical or neurodivergent.

Your child's gifts are sources of energy for positive change. Recognizing and nurturing those gifts will fuel your child's spirit. When that happens, astonishing possibilities emerge. To help you do this, here are some ideas and practices I believe are important, beginning with writing your child's story of self.

Writing Your Child's Story of Self

We all have a story of self. What's utterly unique about each of us is not the categories we belong to; what's utterly unique to us is our own journey of learning. . . . And those journeys are never easy.

They have their challenges, their obstacles, their crises. We learn to overcome them, and because of that we have lessons to teach. In a sense, all of us walk around with a text from which to teach, the text of our own lives.

—MARSHALL GANZ, "WHY STORIES MATTER"

For most parents the idea of writing their child's story of self is something new, and when they hear about it, they aren't sure how it can help. There's already so much to do in the daily routine, why add one more thing? But starting to write your child's story now, and continuing to add to it as they grow and change, is a powerful way for you to connect to your child's experiences. It's yet another way to help you see your whole child and understand how all the dimensions of autism fit together. Your child has a unique journey of learning, filled with challenges, obstacles, and crises that they've overcome already, and that they'll overcome in the future. Exploring that story can lead you, your child, and others who know your child to new meaning and perspective.

You might not realize it, but you've already been building the skills to do this. Just as you've been connecting fragments using a holistic approach to your child's development, you'll approach your child's story by connecting fragments that seem small by themselves, but when woven together become the basis for life-changing insight. If your child can participate, it's essential to include them and allow their voice to guide the story.

Your Child's Story of Self

Generating your child's story of self involves understanding challenges they've faced, choices they've made, and actions they've taken. The questions below can guide you and your child.

If you feel that your child can guide the story, ask your child these questions or modify them as needed:

Think about a challenge (start with one and then repeat the activity with as many others as you like):

What's a challenge you faced?

What was so challenging about it?

Why do you think this challenge came up for you?

Think about a choice you made when facing the challenge:

What choice did you make?

Why did you make that choice?

Where did you get the courage? Or if you didn't feel courageous, why not?

Think about the outcome of what you chose:

What happened after you made your choice?

How did the outcome feel?

Did you learn something?

What do you think others could learn from this?

How do you think this might influence the way you do things in the future?

If you'll be contributing to your child's story or guiding the story, answer these questions:

Think about a challenge (start with one and then repeat the activity with as many others as you like):

What was a specific challenge you saw your child face?

What was so challenging about it?

Think about a choice your child made when facing the challenge:

What choice did your child make?

Why do you think they made that choice?

Where did their courage come from?

How do you think they felt?

Think about the outcome of your child's choice:

What happened as a result of their choice or action?

How did the outcome make you feel?

What did you learn about your child?

What could others learn?

What do you think your child wants their life to be about?

Autistic people have written incredible accounts of their life experiences, and in recent years hundreds of inspiring stories have appeared in books and other publications. In just a few decades, information on autism that was scarce is now abundant, which is wonderful. But it can make it harder to know where to start when it comes to choosing books and articles to read. My suggestion is to begin by browsing. Go to a bookstore or library or look at options online (see my Guide to Resources at the back of the book for a short list of my favorites). When something about the author and their message makes you *want* to keep reading, then keep reading. If you're not drawn in, move on. As you read the stories you choose, don't expect your child's experiences to be the same—they won't be. What you can expect is for the stories to be rich with wisdom that can transform how you understand your child and positively influence the choices you make.

In the rich, textured fabric of these stories of self, one thing is perfectly clear: these are triumphs, not tragedies. This is why autistic people have said they don't feel parents should grieve when their child receives a diagnosis of autism. Instead, autistic people have asked to be celebrated, to be recognized for their gifts, and for society to create space for those gifts to translate into meaningful contributions.

REAL STORIES OF SELF

Aaron, middle-school student, in his own words:

The first time I went to STEM [science, technology, engineering, and math] class, it was so chaotic. It was so bad I even thought about changing classes. I went to the principal's office a few times to tell them what was happening and how other people's behaviors were making it hard for me.

But as the year went on, I got to know some of the kids, some of the seventh graders. Then I started to get used to it. I started to understand. Then it didn't feel chaotic anymore. I fit in. Once I fit in, it wasn't chaos anymore.

I'm glad I stuck it out. Instead of being a rabbit scurrying into a hole, I stood up to the predator. I ate the predator. Eating the predator takes a lot of work. At first I felt frustration, but then I started to feel mixed into the group. It felt great. I felt I had more of a connection, not only with my class but with the whole school.

I learned that I should take my time and not expect to make friends right away. I should take time to learn about the school, the class, and how it all works. I think other kids that are facing stressful experiences, especially if the wires in their brains are mixed up, they should give themselves some time to understand.

Ken, high-school student, in his own words:

Sleep was a big priority for me to do well in my daily schedule, but I had so much stuff to do that it was hard to get enough sleep. It got harder when I started doing a lot of video-related activities, like 3-D modeling, design graphics, and setting up community and virtual events, which I'm really passionate about. I wanted to spend a lot of time on these, but I think it made it harder for me to get enough sleep.

I made a choice to focus on my sleep because if you really want to do what you're passionate about, you need to keep up your health and exercise. I realized that as a teenager getting older, I needed to start being more responsible. Once I did that, it changed how I feel in the morning. I feel more positive and happy. I feel more courage to do the things I'm passionate about and that I choose to do for myself.

I learned that it's not about how much time you spend on an activity but more about approaching it carefully and balancing it with other things that are important like sleep. If you don't, things might go the opposite way and it could all go to ruins. I think I'm headed in the right direction because I'm focusing on being healthy and balancing things, while still doing what I'm passionate about.

I think others could learn that getting enough sleep can make them healthier and happier, and then they can do the things they want to do with more energy.

Nina, mom of fourteen-year-old James:

James lost his words when he turned two-and-a-half years old. Before that, he said words like mommy, up, down, um. He also started losing other skills. He stopped pointing to things. He started to appear lost. He had been a very lively and energetic child before that.

We were told he had delayed speech and to get speech therapy. We did everything we were told but still James couldn't speak. We asked his school if they would teach him how to read and type. They told us not to waste our time.

We felt lost but still believed there had to be a way to teach James to communicate. The therapist taught him PECS [Picture Exchange Communication System] and he mastered it in one session. But we didn't feel that was enough. We believed he could do more.

So we looked for therapists and doctors who understood alternative communication approaches, and they helped us create a program to teach James to communicate by pointing to letters on a letterboard and then typing on a keyboard. We worked with James for hours every day to learn to type. And James made the choice to put in the work. I remember the day when he typed, "I can spell." That was the first magical moment when I felt James was actually here with me.

Since then James has shared so much with us through typing. He can talk to us now just like any other teenager. James tells us his needs, wants, complaints, feelings—both sadness as well as his happy moments—and I think he feels understood. We've come a long way, but still have a long way ahead of us to get where we want to go.

Looking Into the Crystal Ball

Recently, I met with Ben and Leanne, parents of Eric, a rambunctious four-year-old with curly brown hair and freckles. They scheduled the appointment to go over the results of Eric's EEG and blood work and to discuss his progress in therapies. After reviewing his test results and his new developmental skills, we mapped out the next steps of his program and planned to meet again in two months.

Ben had been quiet most of the visit, but as I stood up to leave the room, he turned toward me and started to speak, but then hesitated. After a long pause, he said, "So you think Eric will be okay?" And I realized that in the commotion of a busy day in clinic, I'd focused on the immediate steps of Eric's care and neglected what his parents actually needed most: a way to think about the future.

I settled back into my chair and reached for the laminated visual of the neurodevelopment tree that I keep in each of my clinic rooms. I said, "I feel great about how Eric's doing. You're doing so many of the right things to support him." I pointed to the roots of the tree and talked about all the steps that they were already taking to strengthen the foundations of Eric's development. Ben and Leanne had started meeting with a counselor, who was helping them with the stress of trying to balance work life and home life. They'd enrolled Eric in a great preschool program, and he was in several community activities, including swimming lessons and gymnastics. I reviewed what we already understood about Eric's biology from medical tests and the improvements in his nutrition and sleep we'd seen over the past month. I talked about the development of new brain networks that was happening through his comprehensive developmental and behavioral therapy program and that was the reason why he'd already reached so many goals within a short time. And based on that, I told them I believed he'd be ready soon for even more opportunities in music, arts, and athletics, and that in time he'd be able to explore different academic and vocational pursuits. I believed that his abilities would allow him to participate in a variety of recreational activities, that he'd have strong relationships with friends and family, and that he'd experience joy in all these things.

Ben's expression changed as I spoke. Instead of being preoccupied and distant, I felt he was engaged and present for the first time in the visit. And I saw that Leanne had reached over to hold Ben's hand. Seeing an opportunity open up, I decided to give Ben and Leanne some homework. Before our next visit, I wanted them to write a few paragraphs about Eric's future using these sentences to get them started:

I believe Eric will one day be able to _____

_____.

I want him to have this experience because _____

_____.

I think this is possible because _____

_____.

I can help Eric with this now by _____

_____.

I can help Eric even more with this in the future by _____

_____.

Ben and Leanne emailed their homework to me the very next day. Each had come up with their own responses, and they combined them into a single list:

We believe Eric will one day be able to make good friends.

We want him to have this experience because friends are important to feel happiness and to not feel lonely.

We think this is possible because he enjoys being with people and he likes doing activities with other people.

We can help Eric with this now by giving him opportunities to do the things he loves, like building Lego sets, playing Marble Run, and doing puzzles, with other children.

We can help Eric even more with this in the future by finding more ways for him to enjoy different activities with other people.

We believe Eric will one day have a loving, long-term relationship with another person.

We want him to have this experience because this is one of the great joys of life.

We think this is possible because he's very loving.

We can help Eric with this now by showing and telling him how we (his parents) love and support each other.

We believe Eric will be able to live a healthy life.

We think this is possible because his diet is expanding and he's willing to try new foods. He also loves to be active and has a lot of energy.

We can help Eric with this now by taking him swimming a few times a week, going on hikes together, and taking him to the playground to run around.

We believe Eric will be happy.

We think this is possible because he's already a happy kid! He has a safe and loving home.

We can give him positive statements to build his confidence in his abilities. As a family, we can keep working with our counselor to make sure we're all doing well.

We can help him even more with this in the future by finding ways for him to do lots of things that he enjoys. We can pay attention to any signs of anxiety and make sure we help him with this.

We believe Eric will be able to do work that he loves.

We want him to have this experience because we think work is important, and we think Eric has a unique contribution to make to the world. We know a lot of people who hate their jobs. It doesn't matter to us what Eric does with his life. We just want it to be something he enjoys and something that allows him to give back to others in his own way and make the world just a little bit better.

We can help Eric with this by paying attention to what gets him excited and finding ways for him to do more of the things that interest him and make him energized.

When I met with Ben and Leanne from that point onward, they were much more engaged in thinking about Eric's future. The fear of looking ahead had faded. They focused more on the things they could do to help Eric have the future they hoped for him. And they could see a way to get there.

Everyone has many possible futures. Looking into the crystal ball doesn't mean seeing *the* future, but instead recognizing that there are many possible paths and many ways you can shape them.

THINKING ABOUT THE FUTURE

Here's an example of the "crystal ball" exercise from Marcia, mom of seven-year-old Trina:

I believe Trina will one day be able to have a family.

I believe this is possible because she has a lovely personality and is a loving person.

I want her to have this experience because it is wonderful to have a family and because I want grandchildren!

I can help Trina with this now by providing a loving family experience and helping her develop social skills.

I can help Trina even more with this in the future by supporting her social development and being patient with her.

I believe Trina will one day be able to have a successful career.

I believe this is possible because Trina is very smart and resourceful and has many great interests.

I want her to have this experience because it can be very fulfilling and may allow her to live her life in comfort.

I can help Trina with this now by nurturing her interests and helping with her social and behavioral skills.

I can help Trina even more with this in the future by providing her with more experiences to develop her skills and expand her horizons.

I believe Trina will one day be able to be happy and succeed in whatever her goals may be.

I believe this is possible because she is resilient and strong.

I can help Trina with this now by providing her with support and helping to instill confidence.

I can help Trina even more with this in the future by listening to her and nurturing her goals, but also nudging her in directions she may not understand yet.

Writing Your Own Story of Self

As you've seen throughout this book, the whole-child path is as much about your child's learning journey as it is about your own. Your learning journey as a parent involves not only understanding the five elements of the whole-child path but also allowing your mindset to evolve, especially when it comes to how you think about strengths, intelligence, and neurodiversity. It means questioning long-held beliefs about how you define success in life and what abilities and achievements are truly important. It means looking at expectations you may be imposing on your child based on societal norms rather than who your child is and what matters to them.

As the parent of an autistic child, you're on a unique journey of learning, filled with challenges and obstacles that you've already overcome and others that you'll overcome in the future. No matter where you are on this journey, and no matter what you may think about how you've done, you have lessons to teach others.

At a recent visit, I gave Victoria, mom of ten-year-old Rowan, a set of questions to help her think about Rowan's future:

> *What experiences do you believe Rowan will be able to have one day?*
> *Why do you want him to have these experiences?*
> *Why do you think this is possible?*
> *How can you help him with this, now and in the future?*

She emailed me her answers the following week. As I read her email, I saw that what started as an exercise in thinking about Rowan's future became an act in writing her own story of self:

I believe Rowan will feel loved, develop confidence, and be able to experience peace in his mind and body.

A few years ago I probably would have said I want Rowan to have a successful career, wealth, or high social status, but all those things seem insignificant now. I don't want Rowan to base his confidence on others' acceptance.

It's taken me a while, but I realize that I have to recognize when I'm projecting my insecurities, fears, or beliefs onto Rowan. I sometimes get caught up in expectations and unintentionally project these on him. But Rowan has never fit these expectations, and that's what allowed me to see that I had them in the first place. Now I can slow down and see if my expectations are actually limiting him.

Sometimes I find myself letting ideas about social norms affect how I see Rowan, so now I ask myself, am I looking at him through the lens of his disability? Or am I looking at him through the lens of his uniqueness? Allowing others' ideas to influence how I see him is harmful to our relationship. I've realized that he is an evolving individual, and who he will become is up to him. My role is to protect and support him, which can be a delicate dance every parent must navigate. How do I support a vision for someone who has yet to learn who they are? What's helped me the most is shifting away from imposing ideas and expectations and, instead, consciously choosing to support and be present with him in the small moments of life.

When Rowan was diagnosed with autism, I had to learn how to cope with the fact that I might not have much say in what his future looked like. I felt fear and disappointment because I had so many expectations for his future, even before he was born. I mourned as if a death had replaced him. But now I realize that the *diagnosis was where Rowan and I actually came alive. We were freed from the burden of unrealistic ideas of what childhood, and life, should be. I started approaching life with curiosity and acceptance, and this saved me in hard moments in the early years when I felt like I was drowning.*

Rowan is an amazing human, and my purpose is to support him to be the best person he can be by being interested in discovering who he is, advocating for his needs, helping him tune in to his body and his feelings, and nurturing his curiosity. Regardless of where life takes him, if he has these tools, I'm confident he'll be able to face challenges with the same incredible resilience I've seen in him since he was just a few years old.

If you'd like to try writing your own story of self, you can get started by using the same questions that you used for your child's story of self. Some parents and other family members of autistic people have written extraordinary books that reflect their learning journey (see the Guide to Resources at the back of this book).

Ending Comparison

Comparison is the thief of joy.

—UNKNOWN

From the moment children are born, we begin to measure their physical and mental qualities and compare them with other children. Whether tracking height and weight, developmental milestones, or academic progress, the way we use this information can have both positive and negative effects.

On the positive side, when developmental assessments are used well, they identify areas where your child can benefit from greater support. They might even provide insight into the best teaching strategies to use, appropriate accommodations, and the just-right challenge. They can also tell us when medical tests such as brain imaging, EEGs, genetic tests, or metabolic tests are needed. In this way, developmental assessments play an important role in helping your child along the path toward greater health and learning.

But assessments can also be used in ways that cause harm. For example, children who fall below the second percentile on an IQ test are often given a diagnosis of intellectual disability, a diagnosis that's frequently misinterpreted as the inability to learn. In chapter 4 we reviewed all the reasons why this isn't true. When a diagnosis like this is used to deny a child services in educational, health-care, or other settings, it causes tremendous harm.

Assessments used to evaluate child development are usually designed to compare and rank children in relation to one another. In these norm-referenced assessments, a score is usually calculated as a percentile rank that ranges from first through ninety-ninth percentile, with fiftieth percentile representing the average, or "norm." Assessments sometimes also generate a number called an age-equivalent score. This is a child's skill level expressed as the age at which most children reach the same level. So a four-year-old child with developmental language delay who speaks some two-word phrases and has a vocabulary of about two hundred words might be assigned an age-equivalent of two years based on a language assessment.

Professionals and parents often put a lot of stock in assessment results, but it's important to remember that child development is complex, dynamic, and multidimensional. Children, especially autistic children, have unique developmental trajectories. Evaluating a child's development should always be for the purpose of helping and supporting, not for labeling a child as incapable or limiting their access to services. One of the worst outcomes from an assessment is when it leads parents to feel discouraged or lose hope. Parents who have this experience often decide not to have their child evaluated in the future, and I can understand why. But the answer is not to forego assessments altogether.

Instead, we should de-emphasize percentile ranks and age equivalents and use assessments to understand as much as we can about a child's abilities across all domains of development. We should focus on what an assessment reveals about a child's strengths, rather than view their development through the lens of deficiencies. And we should recognize that children may be growing and learning in significant ways, even when assessment scores don't reflect that. So developmental assessment results should not be the only metrics used to determine whether a child is benefiting from services. The impressions of caregivers and therapists, the results of quality-of-life assessments, and a child's progress toward goals set by parents, teachers, and therapists also provide valuable information.

Comparison sometimes happens in more subtle ways. Children's birthdays, which are occasions for celebration, are one example of when comparison often creeps in. One day I got a phone call from Sue, the mom of ten-year-old Lila, requesting an urgent appointment. It was the day after Lila's tenth birthday. When I spoke to her, it turned out that nothing new had happened—no new seizures, no medication side effects, no worsening of sleep, no injurious behaviors. In fact, Lila's birthday party was a huge success and things were going better at school than they had all year. But Lila's tenth birthday had reminded Sue that her daughter was on a different path than neurotypical ten-year-olds, and this comparison triggered a feeling of crisis.

Comparison is part of our reality—something most of us can't help doing. But when we compare ourselves with others, or our children with other children, we're assuming that one way of being is better than another. Learning to let go of these tendencies isn't easy, but doing so makes room for more joy and more possibilities. You already know that autism brings many opportunities for finding wisdom, but you may not know that *this one*—letting go of comparison—can make the biggest positive difference.

Creating Lasting Change

Though you may not realize it, the steps you take to nurture your child's gifts are steps that also support the neurodiversity movement. The neurodiversity movement strives to create equity and inclusion for people with neurological differences and is one of the most significant global human rights movements of the twenty-first century. In 2006 the United Nations adopted a treaty that reflects how important the need is worldwide. Signed by over 160 nations and regional organizations, the treaty says that all people with disabilities deserve access to all human rights and fundamental freedoms, including the right "to access the physical, social, economic, and cultural environment, to health and education, and to information and communication." You might think that government officials and institutions are best poised to enact these changes, but that's not the case. The changes that will make this possible depend on each of us. Autistic people themselves have led the neurodiversity movement, but all people have an important role in advancing the principles of neurodiversity, especially professionals in health care and education, and you as your child's most important advocate.

The power behind any social justice movement lies in a set of ideas, and the core idea at the center of the neurodiversity move-ment is that differences in neurology and behavior aren't deficits or deviations—that there's no single right way of being. Each of us has our own personal journey to fully understand and accept this idea and to think, speak, and act in ways that reflect it. We all carry im-plicit biases—beliefs and attitudes that are outside of our conscious awareness and affect how we think about and act toward others based on their social group or personal characteristics, like race, gen-der, religion, sexuality, or neurological differences. The belief that typical abilities are superior to autistic abilities is a common bias. Another is the unconscious belief that neurodivergent people are somehow incomplete, broken, inferior, less affected by maltreatment, or less deserving of rights. These false ideas have led to centuries of discriminatory practices and immeasurable harm.

Research on implicit bias shows that it can be reduced by learning to see from other people's perspectives and by learning to recognize and interrupt automatic, biased thoughts. This means learning as much as we can about the thoughts, experiences, and perspectives of neurodivergent people. It also means recognizing when we negatively judge others on the basis of how they behave or communicate, and then consciously choosing to think and respond differently than we might if we accepted those automatic judgments. Once we make these changes in ourselves, we can help others to change. A touching example that we can all learn from comes from Michael McCreary's personal experience in high school, where he experienced bullying and frequently saw bullying directed at other neurodivergent students:

The next time I saw another bully making fun of a special needs girl, I thought I would try a different tactic. Instead of scolding him, I simply explained her situation to him, as clearly and straight-

forwardly as I could. He didn't say anything, but he looked thought-ful. Not long after, I actually saw him playing with her. I figured out that people . . . change . . . if you help them see the other as a human being.

To create lasting change, we need to reshape our own beliefs and attitudes and then help others to reshape theirs. We also need to support reforms to improve the quality and accessibility of health care, education, recreation, and job opportunities for neurodivergent people. The idea that "the personal is political," which became well known during the women's rights movement of the 1970s, applies just as much to the neurodiversity movement today. It means recognizing that the personal experiences of neurodivergent people and those who love and care for them have their roots in social inequities. By understanding and embracing the role we each have in advancing the principles of neurodiversity, we can create the lasting change our world needs.

About Cortica

Cortica was founded in 2014 in San Diego, California, with the mission of delivering whole-child, family-centered care for autism. Today Cortica has a national network of medical and behavioral health centers and a team of over a thousand doctors and therapists—including pediatric neurologists, pediatricians, psychologists, nurse practitioners, speech-language pathologists, occupational therapists, physical therapists, music therapists, behavior therapists, and mental health professionals—all with expertise in autism and neurodevelopment, providing care in centers, homes, schools, communities, as well as online.

Cortica serves as a research network for clinical trials studying innovative diagnostic and therapeutic approaches for autism, ADHD, and other neurodevelopmental differences. Cortica's physicians and researchers have published over one hundred peer-reviewed research articles on genetic and environmental contributors to autism, neural network development, electrophysiology, neurochemistry, metabolism, medication therapies, neuromodulation (device) therapies, and developmental-behavioral approaches.

Family guidance and support is the cornerstone of Cortica's model. From care navigation services to parent coaching, family counseling, and a proprietary online caregiver learning center, Cortica's team strives to empower neurodivergent people and their families to unlock more joy every day.

Acknowledgments

This book has been a labor of love, and I'm grateful to so many people for making it possible.

My husband, Neil, for creating the time and space for me to write this book, for dedicating his own career to turning my vision for Cortica into a reality, and for being a true and equal partner in more ways than I could have ever imagined.

Our children, Kai and Laxmi, for cheering me on through each stage of writing this book and for approaching life's challenges with boundless enthusiasm.

My parents, Dr. Chit-Guan Goh and Annie Yeh-Jin Goh, for giving me every opportunity I could have hoped for in life and more. My mom encouraged me nearly thirty years ago to volunteer at The Ability Center of Greater Toledo and instilled in me a lifelong love of learning. My dad has been my example of a devoted, compassionate pediatrician, always treating his patients with the same care as he did his own children.

My sister and brother-in-law Carolyn Goh and Jason Lee for sharing their experiences as caregivers with me and for reviewing sections of this book. My nephew, Alex, who inspires me with his zest for life and his magnificent mind. My sister and brother-in-law Ying-Ying Goh and Tony Pang for believing in Cortica from the very beginning and being among our earliest investors.

My extraordinary team of friends and colleagues at Cortica—

without them Cortica's existence and this book would not be possible. My deepest appreciation goes to Cortica's physicians, nurse practitioners, medical assistants, EEG technicians, BCBAs, behavior interventionists, developmental therapists, counselors, and members of our administrative and headquarters team, whose commitment to serving neurodivergent people and their families inspires me every day.

Our executive leadership team—Neil Hattangadi, Cathy Lopez, Briana Elvaiah, Ben Nathan, Arun Budhwani, Ipek Demirsoy, and Marc Spooner—an amazingly talented and passionate group of leaders who have elevated Cortica to remarkable heights and filled our journey together with friendship and joy.

Current and past members of our clinical excellence council—Emily Newton, Regina Troxell, Gaurav Yadava, Sora Lee, Marianne Bernaldo, Alann Salvador, Stefanie Canter-Karp, Aqila Armstrong, Antonietta McGuirk, Kevin Shapiro, Elysa Marco, Kyle Gravel, Erin Hafey, Michelle Hardy, Kelly Bermingham, Courtney Olinger, and Kari O'Rourke—who have contributed to the continuous innovation and excellence of Cortica's care model.

Our fearless nurse practitioner leaders, Meaghan O'Dea Johnson and Erin Hildebrandt, who have supported me in countless ways.

Our Talent Acquisition team—led by Steve Harrington—undaunted by the task of recruiting for the fastest-growing company in the field of neurodevelopment, always finding ways to bring dedicated, talented, and compassionate professionals to Cortica.

Our Learning and Development team—led by Steve Ouellette, with workgroup leadership by Savannah Jaska and Olivia Ross—ensuring Cortica's team, clients, and families are learning and growing day by day.

Our Human Resources team—led by Anna Roberts—and our

Diversity, Equity, and Inclusion committee—led by Miranda Sanchez and Christi Eseller—who have championed neurodiversity within our team.

Our Information Technology team—led by Ernesto DiMarino, Sam Roy, and Ambuj Shrivastava—who have built a complex technological backbone to support the delivery of our innovative clinical model.

Our Finance team—led by Ashley Hughes, Antonietta McGuirk, and Luke Hemmingson—ensuring Cortica's long-term sustainability.

Our Operations team—led by Kyle Gravel and an extraordinary team of Area Directors, Marianne Bernaldo, Stefanie Canter-Karp, Dan Diaz, and Lexi Brilmayer.

My special thanks to Cortica's investors—made of friends, family, clients, physicians, and firms—who have supported and guided us at every step and whose belief in Cortica's mission has made all this possible.

I've been fortunate to have incredible mentors and colleagues over the years who have contributed to my growth as a clinician and researcher. My friend and mentor Dr. Bradley Peterson launched my career in autism, taught me to conduct brain imaging research, and gave me unwavering support through multiple stages of my career. Dr. Marion Blank gave me a strong foundation in language development and showed me that nonspeaking children could learn to read and write. Ron Estes opened my world through narrative conversations. Walt Cooper helped build Cortica's foundation with passion and inspiration.

I'm grateful to Toni Robino, soul sister, for her wisdom and heart and for supporting my journey as a writer; Jeff Herman and Marian Lizzi for believing in me and this book; Olivia Ross for creating the graphics in this book with care and creativity; and Sarah Wall for her meticulous research assistance. My thanks to members of the Cortica team for reviewing chapters of this book: Christi Eseller, Miranda Sanchez, Regina Troxell, Alann Salvador, Kyle Gravel, Sora Lee, Emily Newton, Aqila Armstrong, and Erin Hafey.

My deepest thanks to Victoria, Christopher, Rowan, and the other parents and children at Cortica who have contributed so much to my life and to this book.

Guide to Resources

Books by autistic authors offering insights into autistic experiences

Ballou, Emily Paige, Sharon daVanport, and Morénike Giwa Onaiwu, eds. *Sincerely, Your Autistic Child: What People on the Autism Spectrum Wish Their Parents Knew About Growing Up, Acceptance, and Identity*. Boston: Beacon Press, 2021.

Cook, Barb, and Michelle Garnett, ed. *Spectrum Women: Walking to the Beat of Autism*. London and Philadelphia: Jessica Kingsley Publishers, 2018.

Fleming, Jory. *How to Be Human: An Autistic Man's Guide to Life*. New York: Simon & Schuster, 2021.

Garcia, Eric. *We're Not Broken: Changing the Autism Conversation*. Boston: Houghton Mifflin Harcourt, 2021.

Grandin, Temple. *Thinking in Pictures: And Other Reports from My Life with Autism*. 2nd ed. New York: Vintage Books, 2006.

———. *Visual Thinking: The Hidden Gifts of People Who Think in Pictures, Patterns, and Abstractions*. New York: Riverhead, 2022.

Higashida, Naoki. *The Reason I Jump: The Inner Voice of a Thirteen-Year-Old Boy with Autism*. Translated by K. A. Yoshida and David Mitchell. Random House trade paperback ed. New York: Random House, 2016.

McCreary, Michael. *Funny, You Don't Look Autistic: A Comedian's Guide to Life on the Spectrum*. Toronto: Annick Press, 2019.

Mukhopadhyay, Tito Rajarshi. *The Mind Tree: A Miraculous Child Breaks the Silence of Autism*. New York: Arcade, 2003.

Robison, John Elder. *Look Me in the Eye: My Life with Asperger's*. New York: Crown, 2007.

Rowe, Mickey. *Fearlessly Different: An Autistic Actor's Journey to Broadway's Biggest Stage*. Lanham, MD: Rowman & Littlefield, 2022.

Books by family members of autistic people

Cutler, Eustacia. *A Thorn in My Pocket: Temple Grandin's Mother Tells the Family Story.* Arlington, TX: Future Horizons, 2004.

Hammond, Tiffany. *A Day with No Words.* New Egypt, NJ: Wheat Penny Press, 2023.

Martin, Areva. *The Everyday Advocate: How to Stand Up for Your Autistic Child.* New York: New American Library, 2010.

Suskind, Ron. *Life, Animated: A Story of Sidekicks, Heroes, and Autism.* New York: Kingswell, 2014.

Swenson, Kate. *Forever Boy: A Mother's Memoir of Autism and Finding Joy.* New York: Park Row, 2022.

Artwork by autistic artists

Jon Adams, http://www.artspace.co.uk/artists/jonadams/

Maxwell Bitton, https://www.casolvillasfrance.com/magazine/maxwell-bitton-montreal-museum-of-fine-arts.html

Bryn Graves, https://www.saatchiart.com/account/artworks/399322

Jonathan Lerman, https://www.amazon.com/Jonathan-Lerman-The-Drawings-Autism/dp/0807615137

Megan Rhiannon, https://www.instagram.com/petite_gloom/

Mikaela Sheldt, https://www.instagram.com/mikaelasheldt/

Jeremy Sicile-Kira, https://www.jeremysvision.com/paintings

Stephen Wiltshire, https://www.stephenwiltshire.co.uk/

Books about neurodiversity

Armstrong, Thomas. *The Power of Neurodiversity.* Cambridge, MA: Da Capo Press, 2010.

Donvan, John, and Caren Zucker. *In a Different Key: The Story of Autism.* New York: Crown, 2016.

Silberman, Steve. *NeuroTribes: The Legacy of Autism and the Future of Neurodiversity.* New York: Avery, 2015.

Singer, Judy. *Neurodiversity: The Birth of an Idea.* Lexington, KY: n.p., 2017.

Books by professionals
(for anyone looking to dive deeper into topics covered in this book)

Baron-Cohen, Simon. *The Pattern Seekers: How Autism Drives Human Invention.* New York: Basic Books, 2020.

Donnellan, Anne M., and Martha R. Leary. *Movement Differences and Diversity in Autism: Appreciating and Accommodating People with Communication and Behavior Challenges.* Movin on Series. Madison, WI: DRI Press, 1995.

Gardner, Howard. *Multiple Intelligences: New Horizons.* Completely rev. and updated. ed. New York: Basic Books, 2006.

Grandin, Temple. *Visual Thinking: The Hidden Gifts of People Who Think in Pictures, Patterns, and Abstractions.* New York: Riverhead Books, 2022.

Hanson, Rick. *Hardwiring Happiness: The New Brain Science of Contentment, Calm, and Confidence.* New York: Harmony Books, 2013.

Kabat-Zinn, Jon. *Full Catastrophe Living: Using the Wisdom of Your Body and Mind to Face Stress, Pain, and Illness.* Revised and updated ed. New York: Bantam Books (trade paperback), 2013.

Katz, Terry, and Beth A. Malow. *Solving Sleep Problems in Children with Autism Spectrum Disorders: A Guide for Frazzled Families.* Bethesda, MD: Woodbine House, 2014.

Kranowitz, Carol Stock. *The Out-of-Sync Child: Recognizing and Coping with Sensory Processing Differences.* 3rd ed. New York: TarcherPerigee, 2022.

Miller, L. J., D. A. Fuller, and J. Roetenberg. *Sensational Kids: Hope and Help for Children with Sensory Processing Disorder.* Revised ed. New York: Penguin Random House, 2014.

Prizant, Barry M., and Thomas Fields-Meyer. *Uniquely Human: A Different Way of Seeing Autism.* New York: Simon & Schuster, 2015.

White, Michael. *Maps of Narrative Practice.* New York: W. W. Norton, 2007.

White, Michael, and David Denborough. *Narrative Practice: Continuing the Conversations.* New York: W. W. Norton, 2011.

Films

Autism Research Institute. "37 Movies Featuring Autism." https://www.autism .org/autism-movies/.

Donvan, John, and Caren Zucker, dirs. *In a Different Key.* PBS, 2022. https:// www.inadifferentkeythemovie.com/.

Jackson, Mick, dir. *Temple Grandin*. HBO, 2010. https://www.hbo.com/movies
/temple-grandin, https://www.amazon.com/Temple-Grandin-Claire-Danes
/dp/B003ZUTVJS.

Kim, Sue, dir. *The Speed Cubers*. Netflix, 2020. https://www.netflix.com/title
/81092143.

Sproutflix. A collection of films featuring neurodivergent people. https://sprout
flix.org/.

Resources for siblings

Autism in My Family: A Journal for Siblings of Children with ASD by Sandra
Tucker: This interactive workbook introduces the experience of autism, contains activities to help siblings identify their differences and strengthen relationships, and explores how children can understand and support their siblings
with autism.

*Everybody Is Different: A Book for Young People Who Have Brothers or Sisters
with Autism* by Fiona Bleach: This book gives answers to the many questions
brothers and sisters have about their autistic siblings, explaining in basic terms
the characteristics of autism and providing suggestions for making family life
more fun and comfortable for everyone.

Grand Valley State University START Project Sibling Box (https://www.gvsu
.edu/autismcenter/resources-for-siblings-356.htm): This all-in-one set of printable and electronic materials was designed for families to use with siblings of
autistic children and includes conversation starters, kid-friendly recipes, activities, and games.

My Brother Charlie by Holly Robinson Peete and Ryan Elizabeth Peete: This
book explores a sister's view of her brother with autism, the challenges their
family faces, and their journey toward love, patience, and understanding.

Organization for Autism Research (https://researchautism.org/?s=sibling):
The sibling section of this organization's newsfeed contains information and
resources for neurotypical siblings of autistic children, along with first-person
accounts from those who have siblings with autism.

Sesame Street's **Autism Community** (https://sesamestreetincommunities.org
/topics/autism): This website features printable resources and videos designed
to help children understand more about their autistic siblings.

Sibling Leadership Network (https://siblingleadership.org): This organization provides siblings of individuals with disabilities the information, support, and tools to advocate with their brothers and sisters and to promote the issues important to them and their entire families.

Sibling Support Project (https://siblingsupport.org): This organization is dedicated to recognizing, promoting, and addressing the lifelong and ever-changing concerns of millions of siblings of people with developmental, health, and mental health concerns.

Siblings of Autism (https://siblingsofautism.org): This organization is dedicated to supporting the siblings of individuals on the autism spectrum through scholarships, respite funds, resources, and outreach programs.

Since We're Friends: An Autism Picture Book by Celeste Shally: This book explores a friendship between an autistic child and a neurotypical child and describes how understanding and compassion can change frustration into excitement.

Glossary of Medical Terms

Alexithymia
Difficulty identifying, describing, and expressing emotions.

Amygdala
A brain structure involved in the experience of emotions.

Anxiety
A condition characterized by worry, nervousness, or fear to a degree that interferes with daily activities, often accompanied by shortness of breath, a racing heart, or a general feeling of discomfort and unease in the body.

Apraxia or Dyspraxia
Difficulty planning and executing sequences of movements.

Apraxia of Speech
Difficulty planning and executing sequences of movements of the mouth, tongue, lips, and palate needed for speech.

Association Cortices
Brain regions involved in higher processing of information and influencing perception, movement, and other functions.

Attention Deficit Hyperactivity Disorder (ADHD)
A condition characterized by symptoms including hyperactivity, difficulty focusing, impulsive behavior, and challenges with executive functions including staying organized, managing time efficiently, prioritizing tasks, and making decisions.

Auditory Cortex
Brain region in the temporal lobe that processes sounds.

Auditory Processing
The brain's processing of sound.

Autonomic Nervous System

Part of the nervous system that regulates our internal organs, including our heart, lungs, and digestive system, and controls functions including our heart rate, breathing, and digestion. Consists of the sympathetic branch and parasympathetic branch.

Axons

The long, threadlike part of a neuron (nerve cell).

Biofeedback

A form of therapy that uses technology to measure biological activity, like breathing, heart rate, sweat gland activity, muscle contraction, temperature, or the brain's electrical activity, and uses that information to help a person alter their biological activity.

Brain Malformation

A part of the brain that formed differently during fetal development.

Brainstem

A part of the brain that connects the brain to the spinal cord and plays an important role in functions such as breathing, heart rate, sleep, and consciousness.

Cerebellum

A part of the brain located near the back of the skull that's involved in the control of movements, thoughts, and emotions.

Cerebral Cortex

The outer surface of the cerebrum, with intricate folds, that integrates information flowing through the nervous system.

Cerebrum

The largest part of the brain—separated into right and left hemispheres—responsible for managing our senses, emotions, thoughts, movements, and language.

Chromosomal Microarray Analysis

A genetic test that looks at a person's chromosomes for any missing pieces (deletions) or extra pieces (duplications).

Cognitive Control

A mental ability driven by the prefrontal cortex that enables a person to control their thoughts and behavior rather than respond in automatic or impulsive ways.

Constipation

A condition typically characterized by fewer than three bowel movements per week.

Co-occurring Feature

Anything that's not captured in the two core categories of autistic features but happens more frequently in autistic than in non-autistic people. Co-occurring features include a range of medical, developmental, behavioral, and mental health features.

Corticospinal Tract and Peripheral Nerves

Elements of the nervous system that carry information between the brain and muscles.

Cranial Electrotherapy Stimulation (CES)

A type of therapy using a device that delivers a small electrical current through electrodes placed on the ears, which influences the activity of nerves including the vagus nerve and other cranial nerves.

Depression

A condition characterized by persistent feelings of sadness, hopelessness, low self-esteem, and not fitting in, which may result in sleeping too little or too much, low energy, irritability, reduced enjoyment in activities, difficulty concentrating, anxiety, and changes in appetite.

Developmental Coordination Disorder (DCD) or Developmental Dyspraxia

A condition characterized by difficulty coordinating movements, resulting in clumsy, slower, and/or less accurate movements.

Diarrhea

A condition characterized by loose, watery bowel movements several times a day.

Dopamine

A neurotransmitter (brain chemical) involved in many important body functions, including movement, memory, feelings of reward, and motivation.

Electroencephalogram (EEG)

A noninvasive medical test that measures the brain's electrical activity and can aid in the diagnosis of epilepsy.

Elimination Diet

The practice of methodically removing foods from a person's diet to assess changes in symptoms or behavior. This may also involve reintroducing those foods and noting any changes in symptoms or behavior.

Emotional Dysregulation
Difficulty regulating emotions, which may be associated with behaviors such as aggression, self-injury, tantrums, or meltdowns.

Enteric Nervous System
A division of the autonomic nervous system. This web of neurons controls the function of the gastrointestinal tract and communicates with the brain.

Epigenetics
A term that refers to the influence of environmental factors on gene expression.

Epilepsy
A condition characterized by recurrent seizures.

Epileptic Encephalopathy
A condition characterized by recurrent seizures that leads to disruption of brain development and delay or regression of developmental skills.

Experience-Driven Neuroplasticity
A term referring to the way life experiences change the brain.

Expressive Language
The use of words or gestures to convey messages to others.

Feeding Problem or Feeding Disorder
Difficulty eating, which may include difficulty chewing or swallowing, food aversions, and a limited diet.

Food Chaining
An approach used to introduce new foods to picky eaters by using foods that are similar in color, shape, texture, smell, or taste to foods that a person already likes.

Frontal Lobe
The brain region near the front of the head that controls voluntary movement, speech production, and cognitive functions.

Gamma-Aminobutyric Acid (GABA) and Glutamate
Neurotransmitters (brain chemicals) involved in balancing excitation (increased activity of neurons) and inhibition (reduced activity of neurons).

Gender Dysphoria

Distress or difficulties in a person's social life, work life, or other important areas due to the difference between a person's sense of gender identity and the gender assigned to them at birth.

Gender Incongruence

When a person's sense of gender identity doesn't match the gender assigned to them at birth.

Gene Panel

A genetic test that looks at genes related to certain symptoms or medical conditions.

Global Processing

A type of information processing that directs attention to the bigger picture rather than to the details.

Gut-Brain Axis

The collective channels of direct and indirect communication between the gastrointestinal tract and the brain.

Hyper-arousal

A physiological state of heightened stimulation, stress, and/or anxiety. Associated with activation of the sympathetic nervous system.

Hyperlexia

The precocious ability to read words before age five without being taught.

Hypersensitivity or Over-responsivity

Increased sensitivity to sensory inputs, which may include sights, sounds, tastes, smells, or other stimuli.

Hypo-arousal

A physiological state of reduced stimulation and/or energy. Associated with activation of the parasympathetic nervous system.

Hyposensitivity or Under-responsivity

Reduced sensitivity to sensory inputs, which may include reduced response to pain and other stimuli, reduced awareness of how one's body is positioned or how it's moving, or reduced sense of body temperature, hunger, or fullness.

Interoception

The ability to process sensory information from internal organs, such as the ability to detect hunger, thirst, temperature, and pain.

Ion

An atom with a positive or negative charge. Ions like sodium, potassium, and chloride move in and out of neurons through ion channels in the neuron cell membrane and influence the brain's electrical activity.

Local Processing

A type of information processing that directs attention to details rather than to the bigger picture.

Metabolic Disorders

Medical conditions that affect biochemical processes in the body. Some metabolic disorders can cause developmental delay or regression in children and may be treatable.

Microbiota

Bacteria and other microorganisms living in the gut that can influence how a person thinks, feels, and behaves.

Mitochondria

Tiny structures inside of cells that convert nutrients from food into energy that powers all the body's functions and are involved in many other complex biochemical functions within cells.

Mitochondrial DNA Sequencing

A genetic test that looks at a set of genes within mitochondria.

Mitochondrial Dysfunction

A broad term that includes many ways that mitochondria may not be functioning optimally, such as deficiency or overactivity.

Neural Network

Groups of neurons that work together to carry out a specific function, such as a thought, action, or response.

Neurodevelopment

Changes in the brain that make it possible to learn new abilities. There are six major domains of neurodevelopment:

Sensory (how we sense the world around us)
Motor (how we move our body)
Cognitive (how we think, including attention, memory, planning, and problem-solving)
Language (how we understand and use words to communicate)

Social (how we interact with other people)
Emotional (how we process feelings)

Neuromodulation Therapies or Device Therapies

Technologies that deliver electrical or magnetic stimulation to the brain or use software to engage a person in therapeutic activities using a digital platform.

Neurons

Nerve cells in the brain and other parts of the nervous system.

Neurotransmitters

Chemicals that help neurons communicate with each other (e.g., dopamine, serotonin, acetylcholine, GABA, glutamate, etc.).

Obsessive-Compulsive Disorder (OCD)

An anxiety disorder characterized by unwanted and repeated thoughts (obsessions), followed by a desire to get relief from those thoughts by engaging in repeated behaviors (compulsions).

Occipital Lobe

Part of the brain located near the back of the head that processes visual information.

Parasympathetic Nervous System

The branch of the autonomic nervous system that promotes a "rest and digest" response. Activation of the parasympathetic nervous system slows the heart rate, slows breathing, reduces adrenaline, and allows the digestive system to move food forward.

Parietal Lobe

Part of the brain that processes sensory information and receptive language.

Prefrontal Cortex

Part of the brain located near the front of the head that is highly developed in humans and manages complex cognitive, emotional, and behavioral functions.

Primary Motor Cortex

Brain region that controls movement.

Proprioception

The ability to perceive and process information about one's own body position. The sense of body awareness.

Prosopagnosia

A condition characterized by difficulty recognizing faces—sometimes referred to as "face blindness."

Receptive Language

A person's understanding of language.

Reflux or Gastroesophageal Reflux Disease

A condition that occurs when acid from the stomach flows backward into the esophagus.

Sensory Processing Disorder/Differences (SPD)

A condition affecting the brain's ability to receive and respond to information coming in through the senses.

Serotonin

A neurotransmitter that influences many aspects of brain development and brain function, including mood, anxiety, and sleep.

Stereotypy

A term referring to semi-voluntary movements that follow a fixed and stereotyped pattern.

Stimulants

A class of medications that stimulate the brain and may be used to treat attention deficit hyperactivity disorder.

Sympathetic Nervous System

The branch of the autonomic nervous system that activates the body's "fight, flight, or freeze" response to a stressful situation, resulting in increased heart rate, stronger heart contractions, faster breathing, increased adrenaline, and the release of stored sugar to be used as energy.

Synapse

The place where neurons transmit signals to other neurons, which includes the small gap between neurons (synaptic cleft) and structures surrounding that space.

Temporal Lobe

Part of the brain located near the side of the head that processes auditory information (sound) and plays a key role in memory and emotion.

Transcranial Magnetic Stimulation (TMS)

A device therapy that uses machine-generated magnetic fields to stimulate electrical activity in specific brain areas.

Vestibular Sense

The sense of balance and movement.

Visual Cortex

Brain region that processes visual information (sight).

Visual Processing

The brain's ability to perceive and process visual information from the world around us.

Whole Exome Sequencing

A genetic test that looks at over twenty thousand genes to find alterations to the sequence of DNA.

Whole Genome Sequencing

A genetic test that looks at even more genes beyond those included in whole exome sequencing.

Notes

INTRODUCTION

xiv. **one in thirty-six:** M. J. Maenner et al., "Prevalence and characteristics of autism spectrum disorder among children aged 8 years—autism and developmental disabilities monitoring network, 11 sites, United States, 2020," *MMWR Surveill Summ* 72, no. 2 (Mar 24 2023), https://doi.org/10.15585/mmwr.ss7202a1.

xiv. **eighteen others are waiting:** N. Albert et al., "GapMap: enabling comprehensive autism resource epidemiology," *JMIR Public Health Surveill* 3, no. 2 (May 4 2017), https://doi.org/10.2196/publichealth.7150.

xvi. **brain networks and brain chemistry in autism:** S. Goh and B. S. Peterson, "Imaging evidence for disturbances in multiple learning and memory systems in persons with autism spectrum disorders," *Dev Med Child Neurol* 54, no. 3 (Mar 2012), https://doi.org/10.1111/j.1469-8749.2011.04153.x; S. Goh et al., "Mitochondrial dysfunction as a neurobiological subtype of autism spectrum disorder: evidence from brain imaging," *JAMA Psychiatry* 71, no. 6 (Jun 2014), https://doi.org/10.1001/jamapsychiatry.2014.179, https://www.ncbi.nlm.nih.gov/pubmed/24718932; A. Tseng et al., "Using the circumplex model of affect to study valence and arousal ratings of emotional faces by children and adults with autism spectrum disorders," *J Autism Dev Disord* 44, no. 6 (Jun 2014), https://doi.org/10.1007/s10803-013-1993-6; B. S. Peterson, S. Goh, and Z. Dong, "Brain lactate as a potential biomarker for comorbid anxiety disorder in autism spectrum disorder-reply," *JAMA Psychiatry* 72, no. 2 (Feb 2015), https://doi.org/10.1001/jamapsychiatry.2014.2425; A. Tseng et al., "Differences in neural activity when processing emotional arousal and valence in autism spectrum disorders," *Hum Brain Mapp* 37, no. 2 (Feb 2016), https://doi.org/10.1002/hbm.23041; K. Denisova et al., "Cortical interactions during the resolution of information processing demands in autism spectrum disorders," *Brain Behav* 7, no. 2 (Feb 2017), https://doi.org/10.1002/brb3.596;

B. S. Peterson et al., "Hyperperfusion of frontal white and subcortical gray matter in autism spectrum disorder," *Biol Psychiatry* 85, no. 7 (Apr 1 2019), https://doi.org/10.1016/j.biopsych.2018.11.026; J. O'Neill et al., "Parsing the heterogeneity of brain metabolic disturbances in autism spectrum disorder," *Biol Psychiatry* 87, no. 2 (Jan 15 2020), https://doi.org/10.1016/j.biopsych.2019.06.010; B. S. Peterson et al., "Using tissue microstructure and multimodal MRI to parse the phenotypic heterogeneity and cellular basis of autism spectrum disorder," *J Child Psychol Psychiatry* 63, no. 8 (Aug 2022), https://doi.org/10.1111/jcpp.13531.

xvi. **biological basis and meaning of intelligence:** S. Goh et al., "Neuroanatomical correlates of intellectual ability across the life span," *Dev Cogn Neurosci* 1, no. 3 (Jul 2011), https://doi.org/10.1016/j.dcn.2011.03.001.

xvi. **communication for nonspeaking children:** S. Goh et al., "Teaching nonverbal children with autistic disorder to read and write: a pilot study," *Int. J. Dev. Disabil.* 59, no. 2 (2013).

xvi. **whole-child approach:** Anne Brandes-Aitken et al., "Evaluating the effectiveness of a comprehensive, personalized, medically based care model on adaptive behavior outcomes in autism," *PsyArXiv* (Aug 16 2022), https://doi.org/10.31234/osf.io/56px3.

xvii. **"full of health, of depth, of deep human strivings":** Temple Grandin, *Thinking in Pictures: And Other Reports from My Life with Autism*, 2nd ed. (New York: Vintage Books, 2006), xvii.

CHAPTER 1

3. **"how we see things":** Jon Kabat-Zinn and University of Massachusetts Medical Center/Worcester Stress Reduction Clinic, *Full Catastrophe Living: Using the Wisdom of Your Body and Mind to Face Stress, Pain, and Illness* (New York: Delacorte Press, 1990), 3.

5. *co-occurring features*: M. C. Lai et al., "Prevalence of co-occurring mental health diagnoses in the autism population: a systematic review and meta-analysis," *Lancet Psychiatry* 6, no. 10 (Oct 2019), https://doi.org/10.1016/S2215-0366(19)30289-5; J. B. McCauley, R. Elias, and C. Lord, "Trajectories of co-occurring psychopathology symptoms in autism from late childhood to adulthood," *Dev Psychopathol* 32, no. 4 (Oct 2020), https://doi.org/10.1017/S0954579420000826; T. E. Rosen et al., "Co-occurring psychiatric conditions in autism spectrum disorder," *Int Rev Psychiatry* 30, no. 1 (Feb 2018), https://doi.org/10.1080/09540261.2018.1450229; T. Vargason et al., "Clustering of co-occurring conditions in autism spectrum

disorder during early childhood: a retrospective analysis of medical claims data," *Autism Res* 12, no. 8 (Aug 2019), https://doi.org/10.1002/aur.2128.

6. **autism's core characteristics:** American Psychiatric Association, *Desk Reference to the Diagnostic Criteria from DSM-5-TR* (Washington, DC: American Psychiatric Association, 2022).

6. **Some research studies have found autistic girls and women:** M. C. Lai et al., "Sex/gender differences and autism: setting the scene for future research," *J Am Acad Child Adolesc Psychiatry* 54, no. 1 (Jan 2015), https://doi.org/10.1016/j.jaac.2014.10.003.

9. **co-occurring medical conditions:** Vargason et al., "Clustering of co-occurring conditions in autism spectrum disorder during early childhood."

10. **epilepsy and sleep disturbance often occur together:** J. A. Accardo and B. A. Malow, "Sleep, epilepsy, and autism," *Epilepsy Behav* 47 (Jun 2015), https://doi.org/10.1016/j.yebeh.2014.09.081; Vargason et al., "Clustering of co-occurring conditions in autism spectrum disorder during early childhood."

10. **GI symptoms and sleep disturbance:** Vargason et al., "Clustering of co-occurring conditions in autism spectrum disorder during early childhood."

10. **epilepsy and cognitive disability:** Vargason et al., "Clustering of co-occurring conditions in autism spectrum disorder during early childhood."

10. **co-occurring medical conditions between boys and girls:** Rosen et al., "Co-occurring psychiatric conditions in autism spectrum disorder"; Vargason et al., "Clustering of co-occurring conditions in autism spectrum disorder during early childhood."

19. **"If you've met one person with autism, you've met one person with autism":** K. A. Flannery and R. Wisner-Carlson, "Autism and education," *Child Adolesc Psychiatr Clin N Am* 29, no. 2 (Apr 2020), https://doi.org/10.1016/j.chc.2019.12.005.

19. *There is no one way to be autistic:* "About autism," Autistic Self Advocacy Center, https://autisticadvocacy.org/about-asan/about-autism/.

CHAPTER 2

23. **"the uniqueness of each human mind":** Judy Singer, "Neurodiversity: definition and discussion," *Reflections on Neurodiversity* (blog), https://neurodiversity2.blogspot.com/p/what.html.

23. **inspiring stories of people with autism and ADHD:** Temple Grandin and Tony Attwood, *Different . . . Not Less: Inspiring Stories of Achievement and Successful Employment from Adults with Autism, Asperger's, and ADHD*, rev. and updated 2nd ed. (Arlington, TX: Future Horizons, 2020).

24. *Neurodiversity:* Judy Singer, *Neurodiversity: The Birth of an Idea* (Lexington, KY: n.p., 2017).

24. **BDNF:** P. Kowianski et al., "BDNF: a key factor with multipotent impact on brain signaling and synaptic plasticity," *Cell Mol Neurobiol* 38, no. 3 (Apr 2018), https://doi.org/10.1007/s10571-017-0510-4; C. S. Wang, E. T. Kavalali, and L. M. Monteggia, "BDNF signaling in context: from synaptic regulation to psychiatric disorders," *Cell* 185, no. 1 (Jan 6 2022), https://doi.org/10.1016/j.cell.2021.12.003.

25. *experience-driven neuroplasticity:* J. A. Markham and W. T. Greenough, "Experience-driven brain plasticity: beyond the synapse," *Neuron Glia Biol* 1, no. 4 (Nov 2004), https://doi.org/10.1017/s1740925x05000219; K. A. McLaughlin and L. Gabard-Durnam, "Experience-driven plasticity and the emergence of psychopathology: a mechanistic framework integrating development and the environment into the Research Domain Criteria (RDoC) model," *J Psychopathol Clin Sci* 131, no. 6 (Aug 2022), https://doi.org/10.1037/abn0000598.

25. **enlargement in the parts of their brain:** G. Schlaug, "Musicians and music making as a model for the study of brain plasticity," *Prog Brain Res* 217 (2015), https://doi.org/10.1016/bs.pbr.2014.11.020.

25. **meditation show differences in brain electrical activity:** D. Dentico et al., "Acute effects of meditation training on the waking and sleeping brain: is it all about homeostasis?," *Eur J Neurosci* 48, no. 6 (Sep 2018), https://doi.org/10.1111/ejn.14131.

26. **"the rallying cry of the first new civil rights movement to take off in the twenty-first century":** Steve Silberman, Oliver Sacks, and Ebscohost, *NeuroTribes: The Legacy of Autism and the Future of Neurodiversity* (New York: Avery, 2015); Steve Silberman, "Neurodiversity Rewires Conventional Thinking About Brains," *Wired* (Apr 16 2013), https://www.wired.com/2013/04/neurodiversity/.

27. **"No brain exists in a social vacuum":** Thomas Armstrong, *The Power of Neurodiversity* (Cambridge, MA: Da Capo Press, 2010), 15.

27. **not fully human—not whole:** Erving Goffman, *Stigma: Notes on the Management of Spoiled Identity* (New York: J. Aronson, 1974).

28. **shift in mindset:** Barry M. Prizant with Thomas Fields-Meyer, *Uniquely Human: A Different Way of Seeing Autism* (New York: Simon & Schuster,

2015); Jory Fleming, *How to Be Human: An Autistic Man's Guide to Life* (New York: Simon & Schuster, 2021).

30. **a disability and a gift:** Grandin and Attwood, *Different . . . Not Less.*

31. **"neurodiversity-affirming intervention":** K. Leadbitter et al., "Autistic self-advocacy and the neurodiversity movement: implications for autism early intervention research and practice," *Front Psychol* 12 (2021), https://doi.org/10.3389/fpsyg.2021.635690.

33. **Mark Rober shares the story of his autistic son:** Mark Rober, "The truth about my son," YouTube video, https://www.youtube.com/watch?v=ybPg mjTRvMo&t=63s.

CHAPTER 3

35. **"Our differences are our strengths":** Mickey Rowe, *Fearlessly Different: An Autistic Actor's Journey to Broadway's Biggest Stage* (Lanham, MD: Rowman & Littlefield, 2022), 89.

35. **"As long as you are breathing":** Jon Kabat-Zinn, *Full Catastrophe Living: Using the Wisdom of Your Body and Mind to Face Stress, Pain, and Illness*, rev. and updated ed. (New York: Bantam Books trade paperback, 2013), xxviii.

36. **A strength is an ability:** I define a strength as something someone can do that serves them well. A more expanded definition is "emotional and behavioral skills, competencies, and characteristics that foster a sense of personal accomplishment, contribute to supportive and satisfying relationships with family members, peers, and adults, enhance one's ability to cope with challenges and stress, and promote one's personal, social, and academic development." Michael H. Epstein, *Behavioral and Emotional Rating Scale: A Strength-Based Approach to Assessment: Examiner's Manual*, 2nd ed. (Austin, TX: Pro-Ed, 2004).

36. **executed nearly perfectly:** Donald O. Clifton and Edward Anderson, *StrengthsQuest: Discover and Develop Your Strengths in Academics, Career, and Beyond* (Washington, DC.: Gallup Organization, 2001).

38. **Velcro for what's bad and Teflon for what's good:** Rick Hanson, *Hardwiring Happiness: The New Brain Science of Contentment, Calm, and Confidence* (New York: Harmony Books, 2013).

39. **"the 'cannots' and not the 'cans' ":** Tito Rajarshi Mukhopadhyay, *The Mind Tree: A Miraculous Child Breaks the Silence of Autism* (New York: Arcade, 2003), 27.

40. **Perhaps most exciting are the benefits being seen:** H. McClafferty, "An overview of pediatric integrative medicine," *Pediatr Ann* 48, no. 6 (Jun 1 2019), https://doi.org/10.3928/19382359-20190515-04.

41. **narrative therapy:** Michael White, *Maps of Narrative Practice* (New York: W. W. Norton, 2007); Michael White and David Denborough, *Narrative Practice: Continuing the Conversations* (New York: W. W. Norton, 2011).

42. **Repetitive movements:** L. Mottron, "Should we change targets and methods of early intervention in autism, in favor of a strengths-based education?," *Eur Child Adolesc Psychiatry* 26, no. 7 (Jul 2017), https://doi.org/10.1007/s00787-017-0955-5, https://link.springer.com/content/pdf/10.1007/s00787-017-0955-5.pdf.

42. **building on their strengths:** V. Courchesne et al., "Autistic children at risk of being underestimated: school-based pilot study of a strength-informed assessment," *Mol Autism* 6 (2015), https://doi.org/10.1186/s13229-015-0006-3.

43. **If your child processes visual information:** Temple Grandin, *Visual Thinking: The Hidden Gifts of People Who Think in Pictures, Patterns, and Abstractions* (New York: Riverhead Books, 2022).

CHAPTER 4

47. **variety of definitions and assessments:** Robert J. Sternberg and Douglas K. Detterman, *What Is Intelligence? Contemporary Viewpoints on Its Nature and Definition* (Norwood, NJ: Ablex, 1986).

48. **computational capacity within the human brain:** Howard Gardner, *Multiple Intelligences: New Horizons*, completely rev. and updated ed. (New York: Basic Books, 2006), 6.

48. **"Anywhere there are people":** Fleming, *How to Be Human*, 62.

48. **"In a stressful environment":** Fleming, *How to Be Human*, 63–64.

49. **first "intelligence test":** Alfred Binet and Theodore Simon, *The Development of Intelligence in Children (the Binet-Simon Scale)*, trans. Elizabeth Sarah Kite, Training School at Vineland, New Jersey, Department of Research (Baltimore: Williams & Wilkins, 1916).

49. **three key principles about intelligence testing**: Binet and Simon, *The Development of Intelligence in Children*; Stephen Jay Gould, *The Mismeasure of Man*, rev. and expanded, with a new introduction (New York: W. W. Norton, 2008).

50. **"in order to help and improve, not to label in order to limit":** Gould, *The Mismeasure of Man*, 182.

50. **"mismeasure" of human ability:** Gould, *The Mismeasure of Man*.

51. **diagnosis of intellectual disability:** M. L. Braconnier and P. M. Siper, "Neuropsychological assessment in autism spectrum disorder," *Curr Psy-*

chiatry Rep 23, no. 10 (Jul 30 2021), https://doi.org/10.1007/s11920-021
-01277-1; Mottron, "Should we change targets and methods of early intervention in autism, in favor of a strengths-based education?"

51. **different kinds of intelligence:** Gardner, *Multiple Intelligences*, 8-23.

51. **"collection of aptitudes":** Gardner, *Multiple Intelligences*, 22.

51. **"all of the varied human intelligences":** Gardner, *Multiple Intelligences*, 24.

51. **Susan Boyle:** Catherine Deveney, "Susan Boyle: my relief at discovering
that I have Asperger's," *The Guardian*, Dec 7 2013, Music, https://www
.theguardian.com/music/2013/dec/08/susan-boyle-autism.

51. **Daniel Tammet:** Richard Johnson, "A genius explains," *The Guardian*,
Feb 11 2005, Life and Style, https://www.theguardian.com/theguardian
/2005/feb/12/weekend7.weekend2.

52. **how we approach assessments:** Gardner, *Multiple Intelligences*, 167-190.

52. **how we assess children's abilities:** Braconnier and Siper, "Neuropsychological assessment in autism spectrum disorder."

52. **"excellent memory" and "astounding vocabulary":** Leo Kanner, "Autistic
disturbances of affective contact," *Nervous Child* 2 (1943).

52. **savant-type skills:** Darold A. Treffert, *Extraordinary People: Understanding "Idiot Savants"* (New York: Harper & Row, 1989).

52. **Kim Peek:** Fran Peek, *The Real Rain Man: Kim Peek* (Dude Pub, 1997).

53. **Leslie Lemke:** Monica Dybuncio, "9 amazing autistic artists with savant
syndrome," CBS News (Apr 3 2012), https://www.cbsnews.com/media/9
-amazing-autistic-artists-with-savant-syndrome/.

53. **Derek Paravicini:** "Derek Paravicini's extraordinary gift," *60 Minutes*,
Mar 12 2010, CBS, https://www.cbsnews.com/news/derek-paravicinis
-extraordinary-gift-12-03-2010/.

53. **speedcubing:** *The Speed Cubers*, dir. Sue Kim (Netflix, 2020), https://
www.netflix.com/title/81092143.

53. *Fragments of Genius:* Films Media Group, *Fragments of Genius: Understanding Savants* (2000), https://films.com/id/6092/Fragments_of_
Genius_Understanding_Savants.htm.

53. **special isolated skill:** A. A. Meilleur, P. Jelenic, and L. Mottron, "Preva-
lence of clinically and empirically defined talents and strengths in autism,"
J Autism Dev Disord 45, no. 5 (May 2015), https://doi.org/10.1007/s10803
-014-2296-2; I. Rapin, *Preschool Children with Inadequate Communication:
Developmental Language Disorder, Autism, Low IQ* (London: MacKeith
Press, 1996); B. Rimland, "Savant capabilities of autistic children and their
cognitive implications," in *Cognitive Defects in the Development of Mental
Illness*, ed. G. Serban (New York: Brunner/Mazel, 1978).

53. *The Pattern Seekers:* Simon Baron-Cohen, *The Pattern Seekers: How Autism Drives Human Invention* (New York: Basic Books, 2020).

54. **pattern-seeking engine:** Baron-Cohen, *The Pattern Seekers*, 14.

54. **Systemizing Quotient–Revised:** S. Wheelwright et al., *Systemizing Quotient–Revised* (Washington, DC: APA PsycTests, 2006).

55. *Autistic Intelligence:* Douglas W. Maynard and Jason Turowetz, *Autistic Intelligence: Interaction, Individuality, and the Challenges of Diagnosis* (Chicago: University of Chicago Press, 2022).

55. **spins while looking at a rotating fan:** Mukhopadhyay, *The Mind Tree.*

55. **"Woof!":** John Elder Robison, *Look Me in the Eye: My Life with Asperger's* (New York: Crown, 2007), 194.

55. **"cupping our ears":** Naoki Higashida, *The Reason I Jump: The Inner Voice of a Thirteen-Year-Old Boy with Autism*, trans. K. A. Yoshida and David Mitchell, trade paperback ed. (New York: Random House, 2016), 51.

56. **"I do understand things":** Higashida, *The Reason I Jump*, 10.

56. **"I work with data points":** Fleming, *How to Be Human*, 60.

56. **"I have to scan the whole thing":** Fleming, *How to Be Human*, 61.

57. **"Emotions seem to be happening":** Fleming, *How to Be Human*, 74.

57. **"Having a reaction":** Fleming, *How to Be Human*, 40.

58. **some are skipped entirely:** Mottron, "Should we change targets and methods of early intervention in autism, in favor of a strengths-based education?"

58. **Comprehension of complex written material:** J. M. Dynia et al., "Comparing children with ASD and their peers' growth in print knowledge," *J Autism Dev Disord* 46, no. 7 (Jul 2016), https://doi.org/10.1007/s10803-016-2790-9; E. Lanter et al., "Emergent literacy in children with autism: an exploration of developmental and contextual dynamic processes," *Lang Speech Hear Serv Sch* 43, no. 3 (Jul 2012), https://doi.org/10.1044/0161-1461(2012/10-0083); M. Lennox, M. F. Westerveld, and D. Trembath, "Evaluating the effectiveness of PrepSTART for promoting oral language and emergent literacy skills in disadvantaged preparatory students," *Int J Speech Lang Pathol* 20, no. 2 (Apr 2018), https://doi.org/10.1080/17549507.2016.1229030.

58. **Hyperlexia:** Mottron, "Should we change targets and methods of early intervention in autism, in favor of a strengths-based education?"; L. Mottron, A. Ostrolenk, and D. Gagnon, "In prototypical autism, the genetic ability to learn language is triggered by structured information, not only by exposure to oral language," *Genes (Basel)* 12, no. 8 (Jul 22 2021), https://doi.org/10.3390/genes12081112.

59. **"just-right challenge":** E. Dunkerley, L. Tickle-Degnen, and W. J. Coster,

"Therapist-child interaction in the middle minutes of sensory integration treatment," *Am J Occup Ther* 51, no. 10 (Nov–Dec 1997), https://doi.org /10.5014/ajot.51.10.799, https://research.aota.org/ajot/article-abstract /51/10/799/8550/Therapist-Child-Interaction-in-the-Middle-Minutes?re directedFrom=fulltext; E. Kilroy, L. Aziz-Zadeh, and S. Cermak, "Ayres theories of autism and sensory integration revisited: What contemporary neuroscience has to say," *Brain Sci* 9, no. 3 (Mar 21 2019), https://doi.org /10.3390/brainsci9030068; S. J. Lane et al., "Neural foundations of Ayres Sensory Integration®," *Brain Sci* 9, no. 7 (Jun 28 2019), https://doi.org/10 .3390/brainsci9070153; R. C. Schaaf and L. J. Miller, "Occupational therapy using a sensory integrative approach for children with developmental disabilities," *Ment Retard Dev Disabil Res Rev* 11, no. 2 (2005), https://doi.org/10.1002/mrdd.20067.

59. **"optimum-for-growth situation":** A. Jean Ayres, *Sensory Integration and Learning Disorders* (Los Angeles: Western Psychological Services, 1972), 257.

CHAPTER 5

68. **delays like this in medical care for autism:** J. Locke et al., "Parent perceptions about communicating with providers regarding early autism concerns," *Pediatrics* 145, no. suppl 1 (Apr 2020), https://doi.org/10.1542 /peds.2019-1895J.

68. **The wait for an autism diagnostic evaluation:** Albert et al., "GapMap: enabling comprehensive autism resource epidemiology"; J. Daniels et al., "The GapMap project: a mobile surveillance system to map diagnosed autism cases and gaps in autism services globally," *Mol Autism* 8 (2017), https://doi.org/10.1186/s13229-017-0163-7.

68. **autism care is fragmented:** A. Brewer, " 'We were on our own': mothers' experiences navigating the fragmented system of professional care for autism," *Soc Sci Med* 215 (Oct 2018), https://doi.org/10.1016/j.socscimed .2018.08.039.

69. **Clear management protocols:** J. L. Saver, "Time is brain—quantified," *Stroke* 37, no. 1 (Jan 2006), https://doi.org/10.1161/01.STR.00001969 57.55928.ab; M. Stempniak, "TIME IS BRAIN pioneers hope mobile stroke unit will help save lives and dollars," *Hosp Health Netw* 89, no. 1 (Jan 2015).

70. **biological subgroups:** J. Chen et al., "Dysfunction of the auditory brainstem as a neurophysiology subtype of autism spectrum disorder," *Front Neurosci* 15 (2021), https://doi.org/10.3389/fnins.2021.637079; Goh et

al., "Mitochondrial dysfunction as a neurobiological subtype of autism spectrum disorder: evidence from brain imaging"; A. E. Lane, C. A. Molloy, and S. L. Bishop, "Classification of children with autism spectrum disorder by sensory subtype: a case for sensory-based phenotypes," *Autism Res* 7, no. 3 (Jun 2014), https://doi.org/10.1002/aur.1368; M. V. Lombardo et al., "Default mode-visual network hypoconnectivity in an autism subtype with pronounced social visual engagement difficulties," *Elife* 8 (Dec 17 2019), https://doi.org/10.7554/eLife.47427; Y. Luo et al., "A multidimensional precision medicine approach identifies an autism subtype characterized by dyslipidemia," *Nat Med* 26, no. 9 (Sep 2020), https://doi.org/10.1038/s41591-020-1007-0, https://www.nature.com/articles/s41591-020-1007-0; C. J. McDougle, "Another step toward defining an immune-mediated subtype of autism spectrum disorder," *JAMA Netw Open* 1, no. 2 (Jun 1 2018), https://doi.org/10.1001/jamanetworkopen.2018.0280; A. M. Neumeyer, R. P. Thom, and C. J. McDougle, "A rational pharmacologic approach toward a biologically meaningful subtype of autism spectrum disorder," *J Pediatr (Rio J)* 97, no. 1 (Jan–Feb 2021), https://doi.org/10.1016/j.jped.2020.05.001; T. C. Theoharides, "Is a subtype of autism an allergy of the brain?," *Clin Ther* 35, no. 5 (May 2013), https://doi.org/10.1016/j.clinthera.2013.04.009; R. P. Thom et al., "Beyond the brain: a multi-system inflammatory subtype of autism spectrum disorder," *Psychopharmacology (Berl)* 236, no. 10 (Oct 2019), https://doi.org/10.1007/s00213-019-05280-6; Vargason et al., "Clustering of co-occurring conditions in autism spectrum disorder during early childhood: a retrospective analysis of medical claims data."; M. M. Y. Waye and H. Y. Cheng, "Genetics and epigenetics of autism: a review," *Psychiatry Clin Neurosci* 72, no. 4 (Apr 2018), https://doi.org/10.1111/pcn.12606.

71. **treatable metabolic or neurological condition:** A. H. Chepure et al., "Epileptic encephalopathy and autism: a complex interplay," *J Pediatr Neurosci* 13, no. 2 (Apr–Jun 2018), https://doi.org/10.4103/jpn.JPN_172_17; M. E. Marquez-Caraveo et al., "Brief report: delayed diagnosis of treatable inborn errors of metabolism in children with autism and other neurodevelopmental disorders," *J Autism Dev Disord* 51, no. 6 (Jun 2021), https://doi.org/10.1007/s10803-020-04682-2; G. Novarino et al., "Mutations in BCKD-kinase lead to a potentially treatable form of autism with epilepsy," *Science* 338, no. 6105 (Oct 19 2012), https://doi.org/10.1126/science.1224631; M. Spilioti et al., "Evidence for treatable inborn errors of metabolism in a cohort of 187 Greek patients with autism spectrum disorder (ASD)," *Front Hum Neurosci* 7 (2013), https://doi.org/10.3389/fnhum.2013

.00858; S. Srivastava and M. Sahin, "Autism spectrum disorder and epileptic encephalopathy: common causes, many questions," *J Neurodev Disord* 9 (2017), https://doi.org/10.1186/s11689-017-9202-0; T. Zigman et al., "Inborn errors of metabolism associated with autism spectrum disorders: approaches to intervention," *Front Neurosci* 15 (2021), https://doi.org/10.3389/fnins.2021.673600.

72. **thirty metabolic disorders:** Zigman et al., "Inborn errors of metabolism associated with autism spectrum disorders."

72. **more likely to have one of these metabolic disorders:** J. Campistol et al., "Inborn error metabolic screening in individuals with nonsyndromic autism spectrum disorders," *Dev Med Child Neurol* 58, no. 8 (Aug 2016), https://doi.org/10.1111/dmcn.13114.

73. **epileptic encephalopathies:** Srivastava and Sahin, "Autism spectrum disorder and epileptic encephalopathy."

74. **genetics of autism:** M. Lim et al., "Recent developments in autism genetic research: a scientometric review from 2018 to 2022," *Genes (Basel)* 13, no. 9 (Sep 14 2022), https://doi.org/10.3390/genes13091646.

76. **gene-editing technology called CRISPR:** J. A. Doudna and E. Charpentier, "Genome editing: the new frontier of genome engineering with CRISPR-Cas9," *Science* 346, no. 6213 (Nov 28 2014), https://doi.org/10.1126/science.1258096; J. Y. Wang and J. A. Doudna, "CRISPR technology: a decade of genome editing is only the beginning," *Science* 379, no. 6629 (Jan 20 2023), https://doi.org/10.1126/science.add8643.

76. **a number of hurdles:** Carl Zimmer, "CRISPR, 10 years on: learning to rewrite the code of life," *New York Times*, Jun 27 2022; Fyodor Urnov, "We can cure disease by editing a person's DNA. Why aren't we?," opinion guest essay, *New York Times*, Dec 9 2022.

76. *chromosomal microarray analysis:* D. T. Miller et al., "Consensus statement: chromosomal microarray is a first-tier clinical diagnostic test for individuals with developmental disabilities or congenital anomalies," *Am J Hum Genet* 86, no. 5 (May 14 2010), https://doi.org/10.1016/j.ajhg.2010.04.006.

77. *whole exome sequencing:* A. Stefanski et al., "Clinical sequencing yield in epilepsy, autism spectrum disorder, and intellectual disability: a systematic review and meta-analysis," *Epilepsia* 62, no. 1 (Jan 2021), https://doi.org/10.1111/epi.16755.

78. **autistic children have epilepsy:** A. W. Buckley and G. L. Holmes, "Epilepsy and autism," *Cold Spring Harb Perspect Med* 6, no. 4 (Apr 1 2016), https://doi.org/10.1101/cshperspect.a022749; P. Y. Pan et al., "Neurologi-

cal disorders in autism: a systematic review and meta-analysis," *Autism* 25, no. 3 (Apr 2021), https://doi.org/10.1177/1362361320951370.

80. **atypical findings on their EEG:** Buckley and Holmes, "Epilepsy and autism."

80. **potential to lead to improvements:** G. A. Ghacibeh and C. Fields, "Interictal epileptiform activity and autism," *Epilepsy Behav* 47 (Jun 2015), https://doi.org/10.1016/j.yebeh.2015.02.025; S. J. Spence and M. T. Schneider, "The role of epilepsy and epileptiform EEGs in autism spectrum disorders," *Pediatr Res* 65, no. 6 (Jun 2009), https://doi.org/10.1203/PDR.0b013e31819e7168; M. Wang, L. Jiang, and X. Tang, "Levetiracetam is associated with decrease in subclinical epileptiform discharges and improved cognitive functions in pediatric patients with autism spectrum disorder," *Neuropsychiatr Dis Treat* 13 (2017), https://doi.org/10.2147/NDT.S143966.

80. **Exercise and stress reduction:** C. A. Hafele et al., "Effects of an exercise program on health of people with epilepsy: a randomized clinical trial," *Epilepsy Behav* 117 (Apr 2021), https://doi.org/10.1016/j.yebeh.2021.107904.

81. **Dietary changes:** E. Desli et al., "The efficacy and safety of ketogenic diets in drug-resistant epilepsy in children and adolescents: a systematic review of randomized controlled trials," *Curr Nutr Rep* 11, no. 2 (Jun 2022), https://doi.org/10.1007/s13668-022-00405-4.

81. **four diets are currently used:** Eric Kossoff, "What is dietary therapy?," Epilepsy Foundation, Oct 25 2017, https://www.epilepsy.com/treatment/dietary-therapies.

81. **Cannabidiol:** V. Franco, M. Bialer, and E. Perucca, "Cannabidiol in the treatment of epilepsy: current evidence and perspectives for further research," *Neuropharmacology* 185 (Mar 1 2021), https://doi.org/10.1016/j.neuropharm.2020.108442.

81. **nutritional supplements that are sometimes used:** A. A. Asadi-Pooya, S. Mintzer, and M. R. Sperling, "Nutritional supplements, foods, and epilepsy: is there a relationship?," *Epilepsia* 49, no. 11 (Nov 2008), https://doi.org/10.1111/j.1528-1167.2008.01678.x.

83. **brain also cleans out waste:** L. Schneider, "Neurobiology and neuroprotective benefits of sleep," *Continuum (Minneap Minn)* 26, no. 4 (Aug 2020), https://doi.org/10.1212/CON.0000000000000878.

83. **"Even a soul submerged in sleep":** Heraclitus, *Fragments: The Collected Wisdom of Heraclitus*, trans. Brooks Haxton (New York: Viking, 2001).

83. **getting to sleep or staying asleep:** A. J. Schwichtenberg et al., "Sleep in children with autism spectrum disorder: a narrative review and systematic

update," *Curr Sleep Med Rep* 8, no. 4 (2022), https://doi.org/10.1007/s40675-022-00234-5.

83. **biological differences:** Terry Katz and Beth A. Malow, *Solving Sleep Problems in Children with Autism Spectrum Disorders: A Guide for Frazzled Families* (Bethesda, MD: Woodbine House, 2014).

93. **quality of their sleep:** S. Frank et al., "Diet and sleep physiology: public health and clinical implications," *Front Neurol* 8 (2017), https://doi.org/10.3389/fneur.2017.00393.

93. **sleep problems:** C. J. Ikonte et al., "Micronutrient inadequacy in short sleep: analysis of the NHANES 2005–2016," *Nutrients* 11, no. 10 (Oct 1 2019), https://doi.org/10.3390/nu11102335.

94. **Melatonin:** H. A. Nogueira et al., "Melatonin for sleep disorders in people with autism: systematic review and meta-analysis," *Prog Neuropsychopharmacol Biol Psychiatry* 123 (Apr 20 2023), https://doi.org/10.1016/j.pnpbp.2022.110695.

94. **Cranial electrotherapy stimulation:** A. Brandes-Aitken et al., "Pilot feasibility study of cranial electrotherapy stimulation (CES) on behavioral regulation in a mixed clinical cohort," *PsyArXiv* (Oct 21 2022), https://doi.org/doi:10.31234/osf.io/q5z4t.

94. **forms of feedback that help shift biological activity:** E. I. Barowsky, J. Moskowitz, and J. B. Zweig, "Biofeedback for disorders of initiating and maintaining sleep," *Ann N Y Acad Sci* 602 (1990), https://doi.org/10.1111/j.1749-6632.1990.tb22731.x.

95. *gut-brain axis:* C. Shin and Y. K. Kim, "Microbiota-gut-brain axis: pathophysiological mechanism in neuropsychiatric disorders," *Adv Exp Med Biol* 1411 (2023), https://doi.org/10.1007/978-981-19-7376-5_2.

95. **GI tract and autism:** M. Madra, R. Ringel, and K. G. Margolis, "Gastrointestinal issues and autism spectrum disorder," *Child Adolesc Psychiatr Clin N Am* 29, no. 3 (Jul 2020), https://doi.org/10.1016/j.chc.2020.02.005.

96. **microbiota can influence:** H. E. Vuong et al., "The microbiome and host behavior," *Annu Rev Neurosci* 40 (Jul 25 2017), https://doi.org/10.1146/annurev-neuro-072116-031347.

96. **introducing certain probiotics:** L. E. Arnold et al., "Probiotics for gastrointestinal symptoms and quality of life in autism: a placebo-controlled pilot trial," *J Child Adolesc Psychopharmacol* 29, no. 9 (Nov 2019), https://doi.org/10.1089/cap.2018.0156; D. W. Kang et al., "Long-term benefit of microbiota transfer therapy on autism symptoms and gut microbiota," *Sci Rep* 9, no. 1 (Apr 9 2019), https://doi.org/10.1038/s41598-019-42183-0, https://www.ncbi.nlm.nih.gov/pubmed/30967657.

99. **celiac disease to be more common:** I. D. Croall, N. Hoggard, and M. Hadjivassiliou, "Gluten and autism spectrum disorder," *Nutrients* 13, no. 2 (Feb 9 2021), https://doi.org/10.3390/nu13020572.

100. **autistic children are diagnosed with a mitochondrial disease:** R. E. Frye, "Mitochondrial dysfunction in autism spectrum disorder: unique abnormalities and targeted treatments," *Semin Pediatr Neurol* 35 (Oct 2020), https://doi.org/10.1016/j.spen.2020.100829.

100. **milder condition called mitochondrial dysfunction:** Frye, "Mitochondrial dysfunction in autism spectrum disorder."

101. **Mitochondrial support:** Frye, "Mitochondrial dysfunction in autism spectrum disorder."

103. **For many autistic people there's an imbalance:** I. Arora et al., "Is autonomic function during resting-state atypical in autism: a systematic review of evidence," *Neurosci Biobehav Rev* 125 (Jun 2021), https://doi.org/10.1016/j.neubiorev.2021.02.041.

103. **tend toward a state of hyper-arousal:** M. A. Patriquin et al., "Autonomic response in autism spectrum disorder: relationship to social and cognitive functioning," *Biol Psychol* 145 (Jul 2019), https://doi.org/10.1016/j.biopsycho.2019.05.004.

105. **beta-blocker propranolol:** I. Sagar-Ouriaghli, K. Lievesley, and P. J. Santosh, "Propranolol for treating emotional, behavioural, autonomic dysregulation in children and adolescents with autism spectrum disorders," *J Psychopharmacol* 32, no. 6 (Jun 2018), https://doi.org/10.1177/0269881118756245.

105. **Alpha-2 adrenergic agonists:** K. Banas and B. Sawchuk, "Clonidine as a treatment of behavioural disturbances in autism spectrum disorder: a systematic literature review," *J Can Acad Child Adolesc Psychiatry* 29, no. 2 (May 2020); L. C. Politte et al., "A randomized, placebo-controlled trial of extended-release guanfacine in children with autism spectrum disorder and ADHD symptoms: an analysis of secondary outcome measures," *Neuropsychopharmacology* 43, no. 8 (Jul 2018), https://doi.org/10.1038/s41386-018-0039-3; L. Scahill et al., "Extended-release guanfacine for hyperactivity in children with autism spectrum disorder," *Am J Psychiatry* 172, no. 12 (Dec 2015), https://doi.org/10.1176/appi.ajp.2015.15010055.

105. **children receiving CES showed improvements:** Brandes-Aitken et al., "Pilot feasibility study of cranial electrotherapy stimulation (CES) on behavioral regulation in a mixed clinical cohort."

106. **alterations in the immune system:** A. Erbescu et al., "Re-emerging concepts of immune dysregulation in autism spectrum disorders," *Front Psychiatry* 13 (2022), https://doi.org/10.3389/fpsyt.2022.1006612; H. K.

Hughes, R. J. Moreno, and P. Ashwood, "Innate immune dysfunction and neuroinflammation in autism spectrum disorder (ASD)," *Brain Behav Immun* 108 (Feb 2023), https://doi.org/10.1016/j.bbi.2022.12.001.

107. **mental health diagnoses:** Lai et al., "Prevalence of co-occurring mental health diagnoses in the autism population."

108. **up to a quarter of children with ADHD:** R. Cohen et al., "Prevalence of epilepsy and attention-deficit hyperactivity (ADHD) disorder: a population-based study," *J Child Neurol* 28, no. 1 (Jan 2013), https://doi.org/10.1177/0883073812440327; O. Kanazawa, "Reappraisal of abnormal EEG findings in children with ADHD: on the relationship between ADHD and epileptiform discharges," *Epilepsy Behav* 41 (Dec 2014), https://doi.org/10.1016/j.yebeh.2014.09.078; M. B. Mahmoud et al., "Utility of EEG on attention deficit-hyperactivity disorder (ADHD)," *Epilepsy Behav* 114, part A (Jan 2021), https://doi.org/10.1016/j.yebeh.2020.107583.

108. **supplementing your child's diet with iron:** R. Granero et al., "The role of iron and zinc in the treatment of ADHD among children and adolescents: a systematic review of randomized clinical trials," *Nutrients* 13, no. 11 (Nov 13 2021), https://doi.org/10.3390/nu13114059.

109. **children benefit from changes to their diet:** N. M. Uldall Torp and P. H. Thomsen, "The use of diet interventions to treat symptoms of ADHD in children and adolescents—a systematic review of randomized controlled trials," *Nord J Psychiatry* 74, no. 8 (Nov 2020), https://doi.org/10.1080/08039488.2020.1769187.

109. **omega-3 fatty acids:** M. Dopfner et al., "Efficacy of omega-3/omega-6 fatty acids in preschool children at risk of ADHD: a randomized placebo-controlled trial," *J Atten Disord* 25, no. 8 (Jun 2021), https://doi.org/10.1177/1087054719883023.

109. **EndeavorRx:** S. Oh et al., "Effects of game-based digital therapeutics on attention deficit hyperactivity disorder in children and adolescents as assessed by parents or teachers: a systematic review and meta-analysis," *Eur Child Adolesc Psychiatry* (Mar 2 2023), https://doi.org/10.1007/s00787-023-02174-z, https://link.springer.com/article/10.1007/s00787-023-02174-z.

111. **Other device-based therapeutics:** K. Rubia et al., "Neurotherapeutics for attention deficit/hyperactivity disorder (ADHD): a review," *Cells* 10, no. 8 (Aug 21 2021), https://doi.org/10.3390/cells10082156.

112. **Many autistic children experience anxiety:** J. Nadeau et al., "Treatment of comorbid anxiety and autism spectrum disorders," *Neuropsychiatry (London)* 1, no. 6 (Dec 2011), https://www.ncbi.nlm.nih.gov/pmc/articles/PMC3809000.

112. **autistic features or symptoms of OCD:** S. M. Meier et al., "Obsessive-compulsive disorder and autism spectrum disorders: longitudinal and off-spring risk," *PLoS One* 10, no. 11 (2015), https://doi.org/10.1371/journal.pone.0141703.

112. **As autistic actor Mickey Rowe says:** Rowe, *Fearlessly Different*, 70.

113. **potential to promote relaxation and reduce anxiety:** K. Hoffmann et al., "The role of dietary supplements in depression and anxiety—a narrative review," *Pharmacopsychiatry* 52, no. 6 (Nov 2019), https://doi.org/10.1055/a-0942-1875.

114. **Transcranial magnetic stimulation:** E. J. Cole et al., "The potential of repetitive transcranial magnetic stimulation for autism spectrum disorder: a consensus statement," *Biol Psychiatry* 85, no. 4 (Feb 15 2019), https://doi.org/10.1016/j.biopsych.2018.06.003; T. Perera et al., "The Clinical TMS Society consensus review and treatment recommendations for TMS therapy for major depressive disorder," *Brain Stimul* 9, no. 3 (May-Jun 2016), https://doi.org/10.1016/j.brs.2016.03.010; C. Rapinesi et al., "Brain stimulation in obsessive-compulsive disorder (OCD): a systematic review," *Curr Neuropharmacol* 17, no. 8 (2019), https://doi.org/10.2174/1570159X17666190409142555; John Elder Robison, *Switched On: A Memoir of Brain Change and Emotional Awakening*, trade paperback ed. (New York: Spiegel & Grau, 2017). TMS is a promising therapy for autism, but researchers are still trying to understand how to use it safely and effectively for autistic children, so they recommend TMS therapy only if your child is participating in a research trial approved by an institutional review board.

115. **depression is more common in autism:** R. H. Wichers et al., "Psychotherapy for co-occurring symptoms of depression, anxiety and obsessive-compulsive disorder in children and adults with autism spectrum disorder: a systematic review and meta-analysis," *Psychol Med* (Nov 21 2022), https://pubmed.ncbi.nlm.nih.gov/36404645/.

115. **Research studies have shown that gender incongruence:** A. Kallitsounaki and D. M. Williams, "Autism spectrum disorder and gender dysphoria/incongruence. A systematic literature review and meta-analysis," *J Autism Dev Disord* (May 20 2022), https://doi.org/10.1007/s10803-022-05517-y.

116. **differences in sensory processing:** R. C. Schaaf et al., "Sensory phenotypes in autism: making a case for the inclusion of sensory integration functions," *J Autism Dev Disord* (Sep 27 2022), https://doi.org/10.1007/s10803-022-05763-0.

117. **because DCD is so common in autism:** S. Cassidy et al., "Dyspraxia and

autistic traits in adults with and without autism spectrum conditions," *Mol Autism* 7 (2016), https://doi.org/10.1186/s13229-016-0112-x.

117. **accurate measurement of movement differences in autism:** E. B. Torres and K. Denisova, "Motor noise is rich signal in autism research and pharmacological treatments," *Sci Rep* 6 (Nov 21 2016), https://doi.org/10.1038/srep37422.

118. **folinic acid (vitamin B9) may improve speech:** N. Batebi et al., "Folinic acid as adjunctive therapy in treatment of inappropriate speech in children with autism: a double-blind and placebo-controlled randomized trial," *Child Psychiatry Hum Dev* 52, no. 5 (Oct 2021), https://doi.org/10.1007/s10578-020-01072-8; R. E. Frye et al., "Folinic acid improves verbal communication in children with autism and language impairment: a randomized double-blind placebo-controlled trial," *Mol Psychiatry* 23, no. 2 (Feb 2018), https://doi.org/10.1038/mp.2016.168.

118. *alexithymia:* E. Kinnaird, C. Stewart, and K. Tchanturia, "Investigating alexithymia in autism: a systematic review and meta-analysis," *Eur Psychiatry* 55 (Jan 2019), https://doi.org/10.1016/j.eurpsy.2018.09.004.

119. **help with irritability:** C. Fieiras et al., "Risperidone and aripiprazole for autism spectrum disorder in children: an overview of systematic reviews," *BMJ Evid Based Med* 28, no. 1 (Feb 2023), https://doi.org/10.1136/bmjebm-2021-111804.

CHAPTER 6

122. **milestones can happen in a different order:** Mottron, "Should we change targets and methods of early intervention in autism, in favor of a strengths-based education?"

122. **requiring these skills may impede learning:** Mottron, "Should we change targets and methods of early intervention in autism, in favor of a strengths-based education?"

123. **learn new information independently:** Mottron, "Should we change targets and methods of early intervention in autism, in favor of a strengths-based education?"; D. Nemeth et al., "Learning in autism: implicitly superb," *PLoS One* 5, no. 7 (Jul 22 2010), https://doi.org/10.1371/journal.pone.0011731; A. Ostrolenk et al., "Hyperlexia: Systematic review, neurocognitive modelling, and outcome," *Neurosci Biobehav Rev* 79 (Aug 2017), https://doi.org/10.1016/j.neubiorev.2017.04.029; M. Virag et al., "Procedural learning and its consolidation in autism spectrum disorder," *Ideggyogy Sz* 70, no. 3–4 (Mar 30 2017), https://doi.org/10.18071/isz.70.0079.

123. **special interest or "enthusiasm":** Prizant and Fields-Meyer, *Uniquely Human*.

125. ***"The employees in different parts":*** Temple Grandin and Richard Panek, *The Autistic Brain: Thinking Across the Spectrum* (Boston: Houghton Mifflin Harcourt, 2013), 25.

126. **London taxi drivers:** E. M. Griesbauer et al., "London taxi drivers: a review of neurocognitive studies and an exploration of how they build their cognitive map of London," *Hippocampus* 32, no. 1 (Jan 2022), https://doi.org/10.1002/hipo.23395; E. A. Maguire, K. Woollett, and H. J. Spiers, "London taxi drivers and bus drivers: a structural MRI and neuropsychological analysis," *Hippocampus* 16, no. 12 (2006), https://doi.org/10.1002/hipo.20233.

126. **microscopic changes to brain architecture:** R. Stoner et al., "Patches of disorganization in the neocortex of children with autism," *N Engl J Med* 370, no. 13 (Mar 27 2014), https://doi.org/10.1056/NEJMoa1307491.

126. **autistic brain has its own trajectory:** D. Li, H. O. Karnath, and X. Xu, "Candidate biomarkers in children with autism spectrum disorder: a review of MRI studies," *Neurosci Bull* 33, no. 2 (Apr 2017), https://doi.org/10.1007/s12264-017-0118-1.

127. **differences exist throughout the brain:** Li, Karnath, and Xu, "Candidate biomarkers in children with autism spectrum disorder."

127. **Neuroscientists have found that the *prefrontal cortex*:** P. Rane et al., "Connectivity in autism: a review of MRI connectivity studies," *Harv Rev Psychiatry* 23, no. 4 (Jul–Aug 2015), https://doi.org/10.1097/HRP.0000000000000072.

127. **blood flow seems to be greater:** Peterson et al., "Hyperperfusion of frontal white and subcortical gray matter in autism spectrum disorder."

127. **differences in how neurotransmitters:** X. Li et al., "Structural, functional, and molecular imaging of autism spectrum disorder," *Neurosci Bull* 37, no. 7 (Jul 2021), https://doi.org/10.1007/s12264-021-00673-0.

128. **overactive in some brain regions:** M. Ernst et al., "Low medial prefrontal dopaminergic activity in autistic children," *Lancet* 350, no. 9078 (Aug 30 1997), https://doi.org/10.1016/s0140-6736(05)63326-0; Li et al., "Structural, functional, and molecular imaging of autism spectrum disorder."

128. **Oxytocin exists naturally in the body:** A. Preti et al., "Oxytocin and autism: a systematic review of randomized controlled trials," *J Child Adolesc Psychopharmacol* 24, no. 2 (Mar 2014), https://doi.org/10.1089/cap.2013.0040.

128. **Medications that influence serotonin activity:** A. Lee, H. Choo, and

B. Jeon, "Serotonin receptors as therapeutic targets for autism spectrum disorder treatment," *Int J Mol Sci* 23, no. 12 (Jun 10 2022), https://doi.org/10.3390/ijms23126515.

128. **imbalance between inhibition and excitation:** R. Canitano and R. Palumbi, "Excitation/inhibition modulators in autism spectrum disorder: current clinical research," *Front Neurosci* 15 (2021), https://doi.org/10.3389/fnins.2021.753274.

128. **differences in its electric activity:** T. P. L. Roberts et al., "A multimodal study of the contributions of conduction velocity to the auditory evoked neuromagnetic response: anomalies in autism spectrum disorder," *Autism Res* 13, no. 10 (Oct 2020), https://doi.org/10.1002/aur.2369; M. E. Santarone et al., "EEG features in autism spectrum disorder: a retrospective analysis in a cohort of preschool children," *Brain Sci* 13, no. 2 (Feb 17 2023), https://doi.org/10.3390/brainsci13020345, https://www.ncbi.nlm.nih.gov/pubmed/36831889.

129. **altered brain mitochondrial function:** Goh et al., "Mitochondrial dysfunction as a neurobiological subtype of autism spectrum disorder."

129. **differences in several compounds in the brain:** O'Neill et al., "Parsing the heterogeneity of brain metabolic disturbances in autism spectrum disorder."

129. **Other studies of metabolism:** R. E. Frye et al., "Treatment of folate metabolism abnormalities in autism spectrum disorder," *Semin Pediatr Neurol* 35 (Oct 2020), https://doi.org/10.1016/j.spen.2020.100835; M. Manco et al., "Cross-sectional investigation of insulin resistance in youths with autism spectrum disorder. Any role for reduced brain glucose metabolism?," *Transl Psychiatry* 11, no. 1 (Apr 20 2021), https://doi.org/10.1038/s41398-021-01345-3.

132. **Common nutrient deficiencies:** A. Bener et al., "Iron and vitamin D levels among autism spectrum disorders children," *Ann Afr Med* 16, no. 4 (Oct–Dec 2017), https://doi.org/10.4103/aam.aam_17_17; H. Mazahery et al., "Vitamin D and autism spectrum disorder: a literature review," *Nutrients* 8, no. 4 (Apr 21 2016), https://doi.org/10.3390/nu8040236.

132. **lower levels of other vitamins and minerals:** H. Altun et al., "The levels of vitamin D, vitamin D receptor, homocysteine and complex B vitamin in children with autism spectrum disorders," *Clin Psychopharmacol Neurosci* 16, no. 4 (Nov 30 2018), https://doi.org/10.9758/cpn.2018.16.4.383; R. Bou Khalil and J. C. Yazbek, "Potential importance of supplementation with zinc for autism spectrum disorder," *Encephale* 47, no. 6 (Dec 2021), https://doi.org/10.1016/j.encep.2020.12.005; H. Yasuda et al., "Infantile zinc deficiency: association with autism spectrum disorders," *Sci Rep* 1 (2011), https://doi.org/10.1038/srep00129.

132. **for autistic children, physical exercise improves:** M. Carey et al., "The effects of a 16-week school-based exercise program on anxiety in children with autism spectrum disorder," *Int J Environ Res Public Health* 19, no. 9 (Apr 30 2022), https://doi.org/10.3390/ijerph19095471; S. Doreswamy et al., "Effects of diet, nutrition, and exercise in children with autism and autism spectrum disorder: a literature review," *Cureus* 12, no. 12 (Dec 22 2020), https://doi.org/10.7759/cureus.12222; Hafele et al., "Effects of an exercise program on health of people with epilepsy"; C. Ji et al., "Executive function improvement for children with autism spectrum disorder: a comparative study between virtual training and physical exercise methods," *Children (Basel)* 9, no. 4 (Apr 3 2022), https://doi.org/10.3390/children9040507; X. Liang et al., "The effects of exercise interventions on executive functions in children and adolescents with autism spectrum disorder: a systematic review and meta-analysis," *Sports Med* 52, no. 1 (Jan 2022), https://doi.org/10.1007/s40279-021-01545-3; C. V. A. Toscano et al., "Exercise improves the social and behavioral skills of children and adolescent with autism spectrum disorders," *Front Psychiatry* 13 (2022), https://doi.org/10.3389/fpsyt.2022.1027799; A. C. Tse et al., "Effects of exercise on sleep, melatonin level, and behavioral functioning in children with autism," *Autism* 26, no. 7 (Oct 2022), https://doi.org/10.1177/13623613211062952.

133. **reducing inflammation:** C. V. A. Toscano et al., "Neuroinflammation in autism spectrum disorders: exercise as a 'pharmacological' tool," *Neurosci Biobehav Rev* 129 (Oct 2021), https://doi.org/10.1016/j.neubiorev.2021.07.023.

134. **Akian Chaifetz:** Christina Ng, "New Jersey autistic boy records teachers' alleged abuse," ABC News (Apr 25 2012), https://abcnews.go.com/US/jersey-autistic-boy-records-teachers-alleged-abuse/story?id=16209626.

136. **some of these chemicals can interfere with brain development:** P. Grandjean and P. J. Landrigan, "Neurobehavioural effects of developmental toxicity," *Lancet Neurol* 13, no. 3 (Mar 2014), https://doi.org/10.1016/S1474-4422(13)70278-3.

138. *When I was first diagnosed:* Michael McCreary, *Funny, You Don't Look Autistic: A Comedian's Guide to Life on the Spectrum* (Toronto: Annick Press, 2019), 18.

139. **sensory perception is already altered:** N. M. Talge et al., "Click-evoked auditory brainstem responses and autism spectrum disorder: a meta-

analytic investigation of disorder specificity," *Pediatr Res* 92, no. 1 (Jul 2022), https://doi.org/10.1038/s41390-021-01730-0.

140. Understanding Your Child's Sensory Profile: L. J. Miller, D. A. Fuller, and J. Roetenberg, *Sensational Kids: Hope and Help for Children with Sensory Processing Disorder*, rev. ed. (New York: Penguin Random House, 2014); H. Miller-Kuhaneck et al., "Development of the sensory processing measure—school: initial studies of reliability and validity," *Am J Occup Ther* 61, no. 2 (Mar–Apr 2007), https://doi.org/10.5014/ajot.61.2.170; L. D. Parham et al., *Sensory Processing Measure*, 2nd ed. (WPS, 2021).

147. tendency to repeat the same: Cassidy et al., "Dyspraxia and autistic traits in adults with and without autism spectrum conditions."

147. eye-tracking technology: J. N. Constantino et al., "Infant viewing of social scenes is under genetic control and is atypical in autism," *Nature* 547, no. 7663 (Jul 20 2017), https://doi.org/10.1038/nature22999.

150. cognitive differences: B. Dirks et al., "Neural responses to a putative set-shifting task in children with autism spectrum disorder," *Autism Res* 13, no. 9 (Sep 2020), https://doi.org/10.1002/aur.2347.

150. prefrontal cortex gathers information: N. P. Friedman and T. W. Robbins, "The role of prefrontal cortex in cognitive control and executive function," *Neuropsychopharmacology* 47, no. 1 (Jan 2022), https://doi.org/10.1038/s41386-021-01132-0.

150. more attention to details: K. Koldewyn et al., "Global/local processing in autism: not a disability, but a disinclination," *J Autism Dev Disord* 43, no. 10 (Oct 2013), https://doi.org/10.1007/s10803-013-1777-z.

152. Difficulty with facial recognition: I. Minio-Paluello et al., "Face individual identity recognition: a potential endophenotype in autism," *Mol Autism* 11, no. 1 (Oct 21 2020), https://doi.org/10.1186/s13229-020-00371-0.

152. Stroop task: V. Bianco et al., "Electrophysiological evidence of anticipatory cognitive control in the Stroop task," *Brain Sci* 11, no. 6 (Jun 13 2021), https://doi.org/10.3390/brainsci11060783.

154. "assuming competence": Anne M. Donnellan and Martha R. Leary, *Movement Differences and Diversity in Autism/Mental Retardation: Appreciating and Accommodating People with Communication and Behavior Challenges*, Movin on Series (Madison, WI: DRI Press, 1995).

156. "just liked the way it sounded": McCreary, *Funny, You Don't Look Autistic*, 14.

156. *Life, Animated*: Ron Suskind, *Life, Animated: A Story of Sidekicks, Heroes, and Autism* (New York: Kingswell, 2014).

156. classified as nonverbal: H. Tager-Flusberg and C. Kasari, "Minimally verbal school-aged children with autism spectrum disorder: the neglected end of the spectrum," *Autism Res* 6, no. 6 (Dec 2013), https://doi.org/10 .1002/aur.1329.

157. **Research studies that track sound signals:** O. Miron et al., "Prolonged auditory brainstem responses in infants with autism," *Autism Res* 9, no. 6 (Jun 2016), https://doi.org/10.1002/aur.1561.

157. **Temple Grandin describes:** Grandin, *Thinking in Pictures*.

157. **as many as 20 percent of autistic children:** Ostrolenk et al., "Hyperlexia."

157. **hyperlexia to be an early sign of autism:** Ostrolenk et al., "Hyperlexia."

161. **social brain has been called a "complex super-network":** R. Adolphs, "The social brain: neural basis of social knowledge," *Annu Rev Psychol* 60 (2009), https://doi.org/10.1146/annurev.psych.60.110707.163514.

162. **advance our understanding of autism subtypes:** L. Mottron and D. Bzdok, "Autism spectrum heterogeneity: fact or artifact?," *Mol Psychiatry* 25, no. 12 (Dec 2020), https://doi.org/10.1038/s41380-020-0748-y.

163. **the *amygdala* has a notable role:** T. Hennessey, E. Andari, and D. G. Rainnie, "RDoC-based categorization of amygdala functions and its implications in autism," *Neurosci Biobehav Rev* 90 (Jul 2018), https://doi.org/10 .1016/j.neubiorev.2018.04.007.

164. *I just did not find babies that exciting:* Emily Paige Ballou, Sharon daVanport, and Morénike Giwa Onaiwu, eds., *Sincerely, Your Autistic Child: What People on the Autism Spectrum Wish Their Parents Knew About Growing Up, Acceptance, and Identity* (Boston: Beacon Press, 2021), 37.

164. *I did not like and was irritated:* Ballou, daVanport, and Onaiwu, *Sincerely, Your Autistic Child*, 36.

178. **Music therapists use the tools of music:** L. Gassner, M. Geretsegger, and J. Mayer-Ferbas, "Effectiveness of music therapy for autism spectrum disorder, dementia, depression, insomnia and schizophrenia: update of systematic reviews," *Eur J Public Health* 32, no. 1 (Feb 1 2022), https://doi .org/10.1093/eurpub/ckab042.

178. **music can stimulate many brain regions:** Schlaug, "Musicians and music making as a model for the study of brain plasticity."

179. **music profoundly influences brain activity and brain structure:** Schlaug, "Musicians and music making as a model for the study of brain plasticity."

181. **Research shows telehealth therapy:** D. R. Feldhacker et al., "Telehealth interventions within the scope of occupational therapy practice: a systematic review," *Am J Occup Ther* 76, no. 6 (Nov 1 2022), https://doi.org/10 .5014/ajot.2022.049417.

184. **more programs are using a naturalistic approach:** L. Schreibman et al., "Naturalistic developmental behavioral interventions: empirically validated treatments for autism spectrum disorder," *J Autism Dev Disord* 45, no. 8 (Aug 2015), https://doi.org/10.1007/s10803-015-2407-8.

184. **knowledge of neurodevelopment:** A. Rajaraman et al., "Toward trauma-informed applications of behavior analysis," *J Appl Behav Anal* 55, no. 1 (Feb 2022), https://doi.org/10.1002/jaba.881; Schreibman et al., "Naturalistic developmental behavioral interventions."

187. *create more square holes:* Elisabeth Egan, "What does a midlife autism diagnosis mean for Matt Haig?," *New York Times*, Jan 5 2023, Inside the Best-Seller List, https://www.nytimes.com/2023/01/05/books/review/matt-haig-the-midnight-library.html.

187. *masking* and *camouflaging:* L. Hull et al., " 'Putting on my best normal': social camouflaging in adults with autism spectrum conditions," *J Autism Dev Disord* 47, no. 8 (Aug 2017), https://doi.org/10.1007/s10803-017-3166-5.

189. **nature therapy:** V. F. Gladwell et al., "The great outdoors: how a green exercise environment can benefit all," *Extrem Physiol Med* 2, no. 1 (Jan 3 2013), https://doi.org/10.1186/2046-7648-2-3.

189. **improves mood and promotes relaxation:** T. Hartig et al., "Tracking restoration in natural and urban field settings," *J Environ Psychol* 23 (2003).

189. **music activates:** Schlaug, "Musicians and music making as a model for the study of brain plasticity."

191. **"My special interest was important":** Paige H. N., "Why my special interests matter so much to me as an autistic person," *The Mighty*, Oct 31, 2021, https://themighty.com/topic/autism-spectrum-disorder/special-interests-autistic-person.

192. **taking part in theater:** Fleming, *How to Be Human*, 109.

193. *When you are acting:* Rowe, *Fearlessly Different*, 16.

202. **A meltdown is sometimes called:** Daniel J. Siegel and Tina Payne Bryson, *The Whole-Brain Child: 12 Revolutionary Strategies to Nurture Your Child's Developing Mind* (New York: Delacorte Press, 2011), 45-46.

204. **different ABA approaches to autism:** Schreibman et al., "Naturalistic developmental behavioral interventions."

206. **quality of your participation:** S. Ozonoff and K. Cathcart, "Effectiveness of a home program intervention for young children with autism," *J Autism Dev Disord* 28, no. 1 (Feb 1998), https://doi.org/10.1023/a:1026006818310.

208. **"Hope begins in the dark"**: Anne Lamott, *Bird by Bird: Some Instructions on Writing and Life* (New York: Anchor Books, 1995), xxiii.

208. **"So much of our hearts"**: Kelsey Timmerman, "CrossFit helped us face our son's autism diagnosis," *HuffPost* (Dec 6 2017), https://www.huffpost .com/entry/crossfit_b_4519961.

211. **"Self-care is never selfish"**: Deborah Reber, *Differently Wired: Raising an Exceptional Child in a Conventional World* (New York: Workman, 2018), 175.

212. *She's my sister*: Economic and Social Research Council, *Adult Siblings of People with Autism Plus Learning Disability—Their Experiences, Perspectives and Future Support Needs* (York, UK: University of York Department of Health Sciences, 2011), https://www.york.ac.uk/news-and-events /news/2011/research/autism-support/.

212. *I decided I was an adult*: Economic and Social Research Council, *Adult Siblings of People with Autism Plus Learning Disability*.

212. **Research studies of siblings**: H. Kovshoff et al., "Siblings of children with autism: the Siblings Embedded Systems Framework," *Curr Dev Disord Rep* 4, no. 2 (2017), https://doi.org/10.1007/s40474-017-0110-5.

212. **Some studies found that siblings**: E. Jokiranta-Olkoniemi et al., "Risk of psychiatric and neurodevelopmental disorders among siblings of probands with autism spectrum disorders," *JAMA Psychiatry* 73, no. 6 (Jun 1 2016), https://doi.org/10.1001/jamapsychiatry.2016.0495.

212. **social support makes a positive difference**: R. P. Hastings, "Behavioral adjustment of siblings of children with autism engaged in applied behavior analysis early intervention programs: the moderating role of social support," *J Autism Dev Disord* 33, no. 2 (Apr 2003), https://doi.org/10.1023 /a:1022983209004.

221. **"get it"**: Prizant and Fields-Meyer, *Uniquely Human*.

227. **moms of autistic children are more likely to have**: S. W. Chen et al., "Maternal autoimmune diseases and the risk of autism spectrum disorders in offspring: a systematic review and meta-analysis," *Behav Brain Res* 296 (Jan 1 2016), https://doi.org/10.1016/j.bbr.2015.08.035.

227. **About one-third of siblings**: J. N. Constantino et al., "Sibling recurrence and the genetic epidemiology of autism," *Am J Psychiatry* 167, no. 11 (Nov 2010), https://doi.org/10.1176/appi.ajp.2010.09101470; Jokiranta-Olkoniemi et al., "Risk of psychiatric and neurodevelopmental disorders among siblings of probands with autism spectrum disorders."

CHAPTER 9

232. **"free appropriate public education":** Individuals with Disabilities Education Act, US Department of Education, https://sites.ed.gov/idea/.

246. **research studies show that volunteering:** F. Borgonovi, "Doing well by doing good. The relationship between formal volunteering and self-reported health and happiness," *Soc Sci Med* 66, no. 11 (Jun 2008), https://doi.org/10.1016/j.socscimed.2008.01.011.

CHAPTER 10

251. **"Peace and joy . . . are every person's birthright":** Thich Nhat Hanh, quote of praise in Rick Hanson, *Hardwiring Happiness: The New Brain Science of Contentment, Calm, and Confidence* (New York: Harmony Books, 2013).

251. **For Michael McCreary:** McCreary, *Funny, You Don't Look Autistic*, 69.

253. *We all have a story of self:* Marshall Ganz, "Why stories matter: the art and craft of social change," 2008, Friends of Justice, https://friendsofjustice.blog/2009/02/18/marshall-ganz-why-stories-matter/.

271. **the treaty says that all people:** "Convention on the Rights of Persons with Disabilities," United Nations, https://social.desa.un.org/issues/disability/crpd/convention-on-the-rights-of-persons-with-disabilities-crpd.

272. *The next time I saw another bully:* McCreary, *Funny, You Don't Look Autistic*, 55.

Index

ABA therapy. *See* behavior therapy/
applied behavior analysis (ABA)
ableism, 28
acting. *See* theater as a way of building
social and communication skills
activities
adult-led *vs.* child-led, 218
arts and music, 246
athletic, 243–45
nature, 246
outings, 247
religious or spiritual, 246
service, 246
social groups, 246–47
alexithymia, 118, 163
antecedent strategies
cognitive, 198
language/communication, 198–99
for self-regulation, 195
sensory-motor, 196–98
to set your child up for success,
193–94
social-emotional, 199
anxiety
neuromodulation therapies, 114
obsessive-compulsive disorder
(OCD), 112
reducing, 112–13
support for, 113–15
symptoms of, 111–12
applied behavior analysis (ABA). *See*
behavior therapy/applied behavior
analysis (ABA)
apraxia/dyspraxia, 116–17, 146–47

Armstrong, Thomas, 26–27
artwork, observing or creating, 190
assessments, potential harm of,
268–71
athletic activities, 243–45. *See also*
exercise
attention-deficit/hyperactivity disorder
(ADHD)
developmental and behavioral
approaches to, 111
diagnosing, 108
hyperactivity and difficulty focusing,
107–08
non-medication treatments,
108–09
support for, 109–11
types, 108
autism plus, 5
autistic characteristics
co-occurring features, 8–10
differences in flexibility with
thoughts, behaviors, activities, or
sensory responses, 6–7
differences in social communication
and interaction, 5–6
gender differences, 6–7
seeing differences as deficits, the shift
away from, 30–31
autistic intelligence
intellect, 55–56
savant-type skills (special isolated
skills), 52–53
Autistic Intelligence (Maynard and
Turowetz), 55

autonomic nervous system
  developmental and behavioral
    approaches to improving
    function, 106
  hyper-arousal, 103
  hypo-arousal, 103
  imbalance between the sympathetic
    and parasympathetic branches,
    102–04
  measuring the function of, 104
  neuromodulation therapies, 105
  purpose of, 102
  self-regulation, 195–99
  support for improving, 104–06
Ayres, A. Jean, 58–60, 177

balance and motion, 143–44, 197–98
Baron-Cohen, Simon, 53–54
behavior
  defined, 64
  masking or camouflaging to blend
    into social situations, 187
behavioral conditions. See
    developmental or behavioral
    conditions
behavior therapy/applied behavior
    analysis (ABA). See also therapy
  ABC framework, 185
  antecedent strategies, 193–99
  Cortica's ABBC neurobehavioral
    framework, 186
  evolution of, 184
  natural consequences, 202–04
  preventing meltdowns and tantrums,
    201–02, 217
  prompts, 194–95, 199–201
  purpose of, 184
  reinforcement, 203–04
  self-care skills, 188–90
  special interests or "enthusiasms,"
    191–92
  to support a child's growth, 181
  various ABA approaches, 204–06
bias, 271–73
Binet, Alfred, 49–51
biofeedback, 94–95, 105

biological subtypes of autism, 70
body awareness, 143, 197
Boyle, Susan, 51
brain-derived neurotrophic factor
    (BDNF), 24–25, 133
brain development and brain health
  altered connectivity, 127
  amygdala, 163
  autistic brain differences, 126–29
  autistic neurodevelopment, 122–23,
    129–30
  Broca's area, 155–56
  differences in brain size and
    shape, 126
  electrical activity, 128–29
  experience-driven neuroplasticity, 25
  gut-brain axis, 95
  major developmental domains, 12
  major structures of the brain, 123–24
  negative experiences' effects on, 38
  neural networks, 125
  neurons, 11–12, 123, 125, 127
  neurotransmitters, 125, 127–29
  prefrontal cortex, 202
  Wernicke's area, 155–56
brain networks
  about the six major developmental
    domains, 136–37
  cognitive system, 150–55
  emotional system, 163–65
  finding therapeutic partners to work
    with, 177–82
  language system, 155–60
  motor system, 145–49
  sensory system, 137–45
  social system, 160–62
  using the "just-right challenge" to
    build, 166–76

camouflaging, 187
case studies
  Abby (sleep difficulties), 91–93
  Andrew (creating experiences in the
    community), 229–30
  Briana (group dynamics in a family),
    210–11

Ella (specialized private school),
235–36
Ethan (school environment
modification), 44–45
Jacob (medical care delay), 67–68
Jessica (therapy modification), 45
Lila (comparison to others), 270
Marshall (sports lessons
modification), 45
Maya, Ryan, and Sean (mental health
support), 218–20
Michelle (integrative health
approach), 40–41
Patrick (hybrid school situation), 237
Tanya, Joe, and Laura (typical private
school), 234
Wendy (social gatherings difficulties),
45–46
Wes (school difficulties), 238–39
celiac disease, 99
Chaifetz, Akian, 134
cognition
cognitive control, 150–53
defined, 150
global processing, 150–52
local processing, 150–52
prosopagnosia, 152
strategies to support
self-regulation, 198
Stroop task, 152–53
understanding your child's cognitive
profile, 154–55
communication abilities
"assuming competence," 154
augmentative and alternative
communication (AAC), 180
strategies to support self-regulation,
198–99
and stress, 48–49
community experiences
arts and music, 246
athletic activities, 243–45
benefits of, 230
creating, 231
nature activities, 246
outings, 247

as the roots of your child's
development, 241–42
service activities, 246
social groups, 246–47
comparison, ending, 268–71
consequences, 202–04
constipation, 97
co-occurring features
developmental or behavioral
conditions, 8–10, 116–19
medical conditions, 8–9, 73–74
mental health conditions, 8–10,
107–15
statistics, 119
Cortica
ABBC neurobehavioral
framework, 186
culture, vision statement, and values,
222–24
history and expansion across the
country, xiv, 275
mission and approach, xiv, 275
counseling, 180–81
cranial electrotherapy stimulation
(CES), 94, 105
crystal ball exercise
Ben, Leanne, and Eric, 260–64
Marcia and Trina, 264–65
culture
Cortica's culture, 222–24
family background's effect on, 225
importance of, 225
your family culture, 221

depression, 115
developmental or behavioral conditions
conditions related to cognitive or
intellectual function, 117–19
developmental coordination disorder
(DCD)/dyspraxia, 116–17, 146–47
sensory processing disorder/
differences (SPD), 116
developmental profile elements,
42–43
diagnosis based on observation, 70
diarrhea, 98

diet and nutrition. *See also* nutritional
supplements
elimination diets, 131–32
expanding your child's diet, 130–31
feeding problems, 99
food chaining, 131
for improving ADHD symptoms,
109, 110
for improving anxiety symptoms, 113
for improving autonomic nervous
system function, 104
for improving mitochondrial
function, 101
for improving neurodevelopment,
130–32
for improving sleep, 93
for treating epilepsy, 81
Differently Wired (Reber), 211
Different...Not Less (Grandin), 23
disability rights movement, 26–28
discrimination
ableism, 28
against people with neurological
differences, 26–27, 271–73
stigma, 27–28
Drucker, Peter, 225
dyspraxia/developmental coordination
disorder (DCD), 116–17,
146–47
dysregulation, emotional, 118–19,
201–02

echolalia, 42
ecotherapy (nature therapy), 189
education. *See* school
electroencephalogram (EEG), 79–80
emotional development
alexithymia, 118, 163
emotional dysregulation, 118–19
irritability, 119
relationship to social
development, 163
strategies to support
self-regulation, 199
subjectivity of emotional experiences,
163–65

supporting your child's emotions,
164–65
understanding your child's emotional
profile, 165
EndeavorRx, 111
enteric nervous system, 95
"enthusiasms" or special interests,
191–92
environment
biological stress, 136
observing details within the, 53–54
person-environment fit regarding
school, 238–39
simplifying the physical environment
at home, 216–17
epigenetics, 76
epilepsy
electroencephalogram (EEG), 79–80
epileptic encephalopathies, 72–73
seizures, 72–73, 78–79
statistics, 78
treatment options, 80–82
equity and inclusion, 271–73
exercise. *See also* athletic activities
benefits of, 132–33
physical activities as part of ABA
therapy, 188
for supporting neurodevelopment,
132–33
trampoline, 188
eye contact, 42

family issues
allowing for individual interests, 209
dealing with family health conditions,
227–28
group dynamics, 210–11
historical institutionalization of
autistic children, 207
home and family as the roots of
development, 214–15
identity wheels, 226–27
the parent-child bond, 215–20
relationship pairs, 209–10
self-care, 211
sibling needs, 211–14

spreading the spotlight, 208–14
vision statement, mission statement, and values, 224–25
your family culture, 221
Fleming, Jory, 48, 56–57, 192
food. *See* diet and nutrition
Fragile X syndrome, 75, 77–78
Funny, You Don't Look Autistic (McCreary), 138
future, hopes for the, 260–65

Ganz, Marshall, 253–54
Gardner, Howard, 51–52
gastrointestinal health
    celiac disease, 99
    constipation, 97
    diarrhea, 98
    enteric nervous system, 95
    feeding problems, 99
    the gastrointestinal (GI) tract, 95
    GI symptoms, 95–96
    gut-brain axis, 95
    microbiota, 95–96
    reflux, 98–99
    signs of abdominal discomfort, 97
gender issues
    autistic characteristics differences, 6–7
    gender incongruence, 115
genetics
    brain-derived neurotrophic factor (BDNF), 24–25
    CRISPR technology, 76
    DNA, 74–75
    epigenetics, 76
    genetic testing, 75–78
    variants, 24
    variants of uncertain significance, 75–76
Goffman, Erving, 27
Grandin, Temple, 23, 30, 124–25, 157

H. N., Paige (writer), 191
Haig, Matt, 186–87
Hanson, Rick, 38
Hardwiring Happiness (Hanson), 38

health care access, 30–31
Higashida, Naoki, 55–56
holistic framework of understanding autism
    neurons and brain networks, 11–12
    seeing your child holistically, 20–22
    visual depiction, 13, 15, 214–15
the home, simplifying the physical environment within, 216–17
hyperactivity, 107–08
hyperlexia, 58, 157–58
hypersensitivity, 138–39
hyposensitivity, 139

identity-centered language, xi, 28
identity wheels, 226–27
immune system, 106
independence, 166
individualized education program (IEP), 232, 240
Individuals with Disabilities Education Act (IDEA), 232, 238
information overload, 4–5
intelligence
    autistic intelligence, 52–58
    disagreements regarding the definition of, 47–48
    multiple intelligences theory, 51–52
    vs. IQ, 49–51
internal sensations, 144–45, 198
interoception. *See* internal sensations
inventions, 53–54
IQ tests, 49–51
irritability, 119

"just-right challenge"
    about, 58–60
    John example (building friendships), 174–76
    Leon example (two-step directions), 168–71
    the "not-right challenge," 166–67
    Tara example (dressing independently), 171–73
    using your child's developmental profile to create a, 167–68

Kabat-Zinn, Jon, 35
Kanner, Leo, 52

Lamott, Anne, 208
language skills. *See also* reading ability;
    speech
    "assuming competence," 154
    childhood apraxia of speech, 118
    expressive language, 155–56, 159–60
    intended meaning, 158
    receptive language, 155–56, 159
    scripting, 156
    strategies to support self-regulation,
        198–99
    understanding your child's language
        profile, 159–60
    verbal skills without speaking, 57,
        155–57
    written language *vs.* speech, 157–58
learning
    errorless learning, 194
    "just-right challenge," 58–60, 166–76
    neurotypical development *vs.* autistic
        neurodevelopment, 122–23
    "not-right challenge," 166–67
    "scaffolding," 59
Lemke, Leslie, 53
Life, Animated (Suskind), 156
Look Me in the Eye (Robison), 55
Lyubovskaya, Dusya, 163–64

masking, 187
Maynard, Douglas W., 55
McCreary, Michael, 138, 156, 251,
    272–73
medical conditions
    co-occurring, 9, 73–74
    delays in receiving medical care, 68–69
    in families of autistic children, 227–28
    as treatable causes of developmental
        delays, 71–73
    treatment approach categories, 73–74
medications
    for improving ADHD symptoms, 109,
        110–11
    for improving anxiety symptoms, 114

for improving autonomic nervous
        system function, 105
    for irritability, 119
    for promoting sleep, 94
meltdowns, 201–02, 217
memory, 151
mental health conditions
    anxiety, 111–15
    attention-deficit/hyperactivity
        disorder (ADHD), 107–11
    depression, 115
    diagnosing and treating, 107
    in families of autistic children, 227–28
    gender incongruence, 115
"mental retardation" as an unacceptable
    term, 50–51
metabolic disorders, 71–72
microbiota, 95–96
mitochondrial disease and dysfunction
    disease *vs.* dysfunction, 100–01
    role of mitochondria, 99–100
    signs of, 100
    and stress, 101–02
    support for improving, 101–02
moments, exhilirating, 251
motor system
    apraxia/dyspraxia, 116–17, 146–47
    brain regions and their roles, 146
    eating and swallowing, 149
    eye usage, 149
    fine motor skills, 148–49
    gross motor skills, 147–48
    relationship with the sensory system,
        145–46
    sound formation, 149
    understanding your child's motor
        profile, 147–49
    voluntary *vs.* involuntary
        movements, 146
Mukhopadhyay, Tito, 39, 55
multiple intelligences theory, 51–52
music
    as an activity within the community,
        246
    music therapy, 178–79
    as a self-care skill, 189–90

narrative therapy, 41–42
natural consequences, 202–04
nature
    nature activities, 246
    nature therapy (ecotherapy), 189
needs and wants, 217
negativity bias, 38–40
nervous system, 102. *See also* autonomic
    nervous system
neurodevelopment
    building brain networks, 136–65
    diet and nutrition for improving,
        130–32
    exercise for improving, 132–33
    family as the roots of, 214–15
    improving overall health for, 129–30
    neurotypical *vs.* autistic, 122–23
    relationships for improving, 133–35
    and stress, 135–36
neurodevelopmental profile, 16–19
neurodivergent, 29
neurodiversity
    defined, 24, 29
    neurodiversity-affirming intervention,
        31–33
the neurodiversity movement
    debates within, 30–31
    educating others about, 31–33
    the fight for equity and inclusion,
        271–73
    identity-centered language, xi, 28
    roots in the disability rights
        movement, 26–28
    as social justice, 25–26
neurological conditions, importance of
    rapid treatment for, 69
neuromodulation therapies
    biofeedback, 94–95, 105
    cranial electrotherapy stimulation
        (CES), 94, 105
    EndeavorRx, 111
    transcranial magnetic stimulation
        (TMS), 114
neurotransmitters
    dopamine, 128
    GABA and glutamate, 128

role of, 125, 127
    serotonin, 128
NeuroTribes (Silberman), 25–26
neurotypical development *vs.* autistic
    neurodevelopment, 122–23
non-contingent reinforcement, 189
nonspeaking, xii, 57, 155–57
"not-right challenge," 166–67
nutritional supplements. *See also* diet
        and nutrition
    for improving ADHD symptoms, 110
    for improving anxiety symptoms,
        113–14
    for improving autonomic nervous
        system function, 104–05
    for improving mitochondrial
        function, 101–02
    for improving sleep health, 93–94
    for vitamin or mineral
        deficiencies, 132

obsessive-compulsive disorder
    (OCD), 112
occupational therapy (OT), 177–78, 241
outings to public venues, 247
overload, 201
overstimulation, 134

parasympathetic branch of the
    autonomic nervous system, 102–04
Paravicini, Derek, 53
parent-child bond, strengthening the,
    215–20
Park, Max, 53, 121
*The Pattern Seekers: How Autism
    Drives Human Invention*
    (Baron-Cohen), 53
pattern-seeking, 53–55
Peek, Kim, 52–53
person-centered approach *vs.*
    disease-centered approach,
    40–41
person-environment fit, 238–39
physical therapy (PT), 179
The Power of Neurodiversity
    (Armstrong), 26–27

problems, 41–42
professional success, 253
profile, understanding your child's
  unique, 16–19
prompts
  examples, 194–95
  physical, 195, 199–200
  prompt fading, 200–01
  using the least intrusive, 200
  verbal, 195, 200
  visual, 195, 200
proprioception. *See* body awareness
prosopagnosia, 152

reading ability. *See also* language skills;
  speech
  hyperlexia, 58, 157–58
  before speaking ability, 58
  visual processing skills, 157–58
The Reason I Jump (Higashida), 55–56
Reber, Deborah, 211
reflux, 98–99
reinforcement, 203–04
relationships, 133–35
religious or spiritual activities, 246
repetitive behaviors, 53–55, 112, 146
research
  innovation in autism care, xiii–xiv
  statistics, xiv
resources
  finding helpers, 220–21
  therapeutic partners to help your
    child, 177–82
Rober, Mark, 33
Robison, John Elder, 30, 55
Rowe, Mickey, 112–13, 193

savant-type skills (special isolated
  skills), 52–53
school
  challenge of tailoring curricula to
    autistic students, 60
  choosing a school, 231
  gen ed *vs.* special ed classrooms,
    232–33
  homeschooling, 236

individualized education program
  (IEP), 232, 240
Individuals with Disabilities
  Education Act (IDEA), 232, 238
person-environment fit, 238–39
public school, 232–33
school-provided evaluations and
  therapies, 240–41
social growth, 239
special education advocates and
  attorneys, 239
typical *vs.* specialized private schools,
  233–36
seizures, 72–73, 78–79
self-care
  for your child, 188–90
  for yourself, 211
self-regulation, 195–99
sensory information
  balance and motion, 143–44, 197–98
  body awareness, 143, 197
  hypersensitivity, 138–39
  hyposensitivity, 139
  internal sensations, 144–45, 198
  meltdowns, 201–02, 217
  and the motor system, 145–46
  overstimulation from social
    interactions, 134
  processing, 58–59
  sensory-motor strategies to support
    self-regulation, 196–98
  sensory processing disorder/
    differences (SPD), 116
  sensory receptors, 137–38
  sight, 140–41, 196
  simplifying the physical environment
    at home, 216–17
  smell, 142–43, 197
  sound, 140, 196
  taste, 142
  touch, 141–42, 196–97
  understanding your child's sensory
    profile, 140–45
service activities, 246
Shore, Stephen, 19
sibling needs, 211–14

sight, 140–41, 196

Silberman, Steve, 25–26

Sincerely, Your Autistic Child
   (Lyubovskaya), 163–64

sleep
   activities to improve, 86–88
   biological processes during, 83
   difficulties, 83–84
   EEG testing during, 80
   falling asleep independently,
     89–90
   neuromodulation therapies,
     94–95
   requirements, 84
   the sleep environment, 88–89
   sleep story, 90–91
   support for improving, 93–95
   tracking worksheet, 84–86
   waking during the night, 89–90

smell, 142–43, 197

social development
   complexities of certain social
     situations, 161
   and its reliance on all the other
     systems, 160–61, 163
   social groups, 246–47
   social growth, 239
   special interests or "enthusiasms,"
     191–92
   strategies to support
     self-regulation, 199
   through theater, 192–93
   typical social practices, 192–93
   understanding your child's social
     profile, 162
   using social interaction to support
     neurodevelopment, 133–35

sound, 140, 157, 196

special interests or "enthusiasms,"
   191–92

speech. *See also* language skills; reading
   ability
   "assuming competence," 154
   childhood apraxia of speech, 118
   neurotypical development, 57–58
   scripting, 156

   and social interaction, 118
   verbal skills without speaking, 57,
     155–57

speech-language therapy (SLT), 180

stereotypies, 42, 146

stigma, 27–28

story of self
   Aaron's story of self, 257–58
   by autistic authors, 256–57
   James' story of self, 259–60
   Ken's story of self, 258–59
   questions for writing your child's
     story of self, 255–56
   Rowan's story of self, 266–68
   as a way of understanding your child,
     253–54
   writing your own, 266–68

strengths
   defining, 36–38
   recognizing, 37–38
   strengths-finding exercise, 37

strengths-based approach
   modification of the environment,
     44–46
   person-environment fit, 42–44

stress
   biological, 136
   effect on communication abilities,
     48–49
   and mitochondrial function, 101–02
   strategies for dealing with, 135–36
   the stress response, 135

success
   antecedent strategies to set your child
     up for success, 193–94
   experiencing, 194
   professional, 253

support requirements, 60

Suskind, Owen, 156

Suskind, Ron, 156

sympathetic branch of the autonomic
   nervous system, 102–04

Tammet, Daniel, 51–52

tantrums, 201–02

taste, 142

telehealth therapies, 181
testing
  age-equivalent score, 269
  assessments, potential harm of,
    268–71
  genetic, 75–78
  intelligence, 49–51
  using multiple observations and
    assessments, 52
theater as a way of building social and
  communication skills, 192–93, 246
therapy. *See also* behavior therapy/
  applied behavior analysis (ABA)
  counseling, 180–81
  for developmental coordination
    disorder (DCD), 117
  for improving ADHD symptoms, 111
  for improving autonomic nervous
    system function, 106
  music therapy, 178–79
  narrative therapy, 41–42
  occupational therapy (OT),
    177–78, 241
  physical therapy (PT), 179
  school-provided, 240–41
  speech-language therapy (SLT), 180

telehealth therapies, 181
  therapeutic partners to help your
    child, 177–82
Timmerman, Kelsey, 208–09
touch, 141–42, 196–97
transcranial magnetic stimulation
  (TMS), 114
treatment approaches for co-occurring
  medical conditions, 73–74
tunnel vision in autism care, problems
  with, 14
Turowetz, Jason, 55

vagus nerve stimulation, 82
verbal ability. *See* speech
vestibular sense. *See* balance and motion

whole-child path
  key elements, 64–65
  the learning journey of parents and
    children, 266
  talents and gifts found on the,
    252–53
"Why Stories Matter" (article), 253–54
Wiltshire, Stephen, 53
written language *vs.* speech, 157–58

About the Author

Suzanne Goh, MD, BCBA, is a pediatric neurologist, behavior analyst, and neuroscience researcher. She is the cofounder and Chief Medical Officer of Cortica—the nation's leading provider of whole-child care for autism. Dr. Goh graduated from Harvard Medical School with honors and attended Oxford University as a Rhodes Scholar. At Columbia University she served as assistant professor of Clinical Neurology and codirector of Columbia's Developmental Neuropsychiatry Center for Autism. Her research has focused on the biological basis of autism, developmental outcomes from whole-child autism care, and novel therapies for neurodevelopment. Her work has led to publication in leading neuroscience journals, including *Neurology*, *Annals of Neurology*, and *JAMA Psychiatry*. Dr. Goh lives in San Diego, California, with her husband, Neil Hattangadi, and their two children.